HPNA PALLIATIVE NURSING MANUALS

# Legal and Ethical Aspects of Care

## HPNA PALLIATIVE NURSING MANUALS

*Series edited by: Betty R. Ferrell, RN, PhD, MA, FAAN, FPCN, CHPN*

Volume 1: Structure and Processes of Care

Volume 2: Physical Aspects of Care: Pain and Gastrointestinal Symptoms

Volume 3: Physical Aspects of Care: Nutritional, Dermatologic, Neurologic, and Other Symptoms

Volume 4: Pediatric Palliative Care

Volume 5: Spiritual, Religious, and Existential Aspects of Care and Cultural Aspects

Volume 6: Social Aspects of Care

Volume 7: Care of the Imminently Dying

Volume 8: Legal and Ethical Aspects of Care

HPNA PALLIATIVE NURSING MANUALS

# Legal and Ethical Aspects of Care

Edited by

## Nessa Coyle, PhD, APRN, FAAN

Consultant
Palliative Care and Clinical Ethics in Oncology
New York, New York

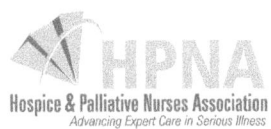

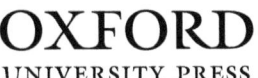

# OXFORD
UNIVERSITY PRESS

Oxford University Press is a department of the University of Oxford. It furthers the University's objective of excellence in research, scholarship, and education by publishing worldwide.Oxford is a registered trade mark of Oxford University Press in the UK and certain other countries.

Published in the United States of America by Oxford University Press
198 Madison Avenue, New York, NY 10016, United States of America.

© Oxford University Press 2016

First Edition published in 2016

All rights reserved. No part of this publication may be reproduced, stored in a retrieval system, or transmitted, in any form or by any means, without the prior permission in writing of Oxford University Press, or as expressly permitted by law, by license, or under terms agreed with the appropriate reproduction rights organization. Inquiries concerning reproduction outside the scope of the above should be sent to the Rights Department, Oxford University Press, at the address above.

You must not circulate this work in any other form
and you must impose this same condition on any acquirer.

Library of Congress Cataloging-in-Publication Data
Legal and ethical aspects of care / edited by Nessa Coyle.
   p. ; cm. — (HPNA palliative nursing manuals)
Includes bibliographical references and index.
ISBN 978-0-19-025806-1 (alk. paper)
I. Coyle, Nessa, editor.   II. Series: HPNA palliative nursing manuals.
[DNLM: 1. Palliative Care—ethics.   2. Terminal Care—ethics.   3. Terminal Care—legislation & jurisprudence.   4. Palliative Care—legislation & jurisprudence.   WB 310]
R725.5
174.2'96029—dc23
2015028361

This material is not intended to be, and should not be considered, a substitute for medical or other professional advice. Treatment for the conditions described in this material is highly dependent on the individual circumstances. And, while this material is designed to offer accurate information with respect to the subject matter covered and to be current as of the time it was written, research and knowledge about medical and health issues is constantly evolving and dose schedules for medications are being revised continually, with new side effects recognized and accounted for regularly. Readers must therefore always check the product information and clinical procedures with the most up-to-date published product information and data sheets provided by the manufacturers and the most recent codes of conduct and safety regulation. The publisher and the authors make no representations or warranties to readers, express or implied, as to the accuracy or completeness of this material. Without limiting the foregoing, the publisher and the authors make no representations or warranties as to the accuracy or efficacy of the drug dosages mentioned in the material. The authors and the publisher do not accept, and expressly disclaim, any responsibility for any liability, loss or risk that may be claimed or incurred as a consequence of the use
and/or application of any of the contents of this material.

# Contents

Preface *vii*
Contributors *ix*

1. Ethical Considerations in Palliative Care *1*
   *Maryjo Prince-Paul and Barbara J. Daly*

2. Palliative Care and Requests for Assistance in Dying *29*
   *Deborah L. Volker*

3. Artificial Nutrition and Hydration *47*
   *Michelle S. Gabriel and Jennifer A. Tschanz*

4. End-of-Life Care for Patients With Mental Illness and Personality Disorders *67*
   *Betty D. Morgan*

5. Poor, Homeless, and Underserved Populations *89*
   *Anne Hughes*

Appendix: Self-Assessment Test Questions *117*
*Nessa Coyle*

Index *119*

# Preface

This is the eighth volume of a new series being published by Oxford University Press in collaboration with the Hospice and Palliative Nurses Association. The intent of this series is to provide palliative care nurses with quick reference guides to each of the key domains of palliative care.

Content for this series was derived primarily from the *Oxford Textbook of Palliative Nursing* (4th edition, 2015), which is also edited by Betty Ferrell, Nessa Coyle, and Judith Paice, the editors of this series. The Contributors identified in each volume are the authors of chapters in the *Oxford Textbook of Palliative Nursing* from which the content was selected for this volume. The *Textbook* contains more extensive content and references so users of this Palliative Nursing Series are encouraged to use the *Textbook* as an additional resource.

We are grateful to all palliative care nurses who are contributing to the advancement of care for seriously ill patients and families. Remarkable progress has occurred over the past 30 years in this field, and nurses have been central to that progress. Our hope is that this series offers an additional tool to build the care delivery system we strive for.

# Contributors

**Barbara J. Daly, PhD, RN, FAAN**
The Gertrude Perkins Oliva Professor of Oncology Nursing
Frances Payne Bolton School of Nursing
Case Western Reserve University
University Hospital of Cleveland
Cleveland, Ohio

**Michelle S. Gabriel, RN, MS, ACHPN**
Palliative Care Clinical Nurse Specialist
VA Palo Alto Health Care System
Palo Alto, California

**Anne Hughes, RN, ACHPN, PhD, FAAN**
Advanced Practice Nurse
Palliative Care Service
Laguna Honda Hospital and Rehabilitation Center
San Francisco, California

**Betty D. Morgan, PhD, PMHCNS, BC**
Associate Professor Emeritus
School of Nursing, College of Health Sciences
University of Massachusetts
Lowell, Massachusetts

**Maryjo Prince-Paul, PhD, APRN, ACHPN, FPCN**
Assistant Professor of Nursing
Frances Payne Bolton School of Nursing
Case Western Reserve University
Cleveland, Ohio

**Jennifer A. Tschanz, RN, MSN, FNP, AOCNP**
Nurse Practitioner
Department of Hematology Oncology
Naval Medical Center San Diego
San Diego, California

**Deborah L. Volker, PhD, RN, AOCN, FAAN**
Associate Professor of Nursing
School of Nursing
The University of Texas at Austin
Austin, Texas

# Chapter 1

# Ethical Considerations in Palliative Care

Maryjo Prince-Paul and Barbara J. Daly

> **Key Points**
> - What constitutes "extraordinary care" is almost entirely contingent on the values and clinical situation of the patient.
> - Enteral and parenteral nutrition and hydration are medical treatments that can be withheld or withdrawn under appropriate medical and ethical circumstances.
> - Effective palliative care that rests on a sound ethical foundation requires ongoing discussion about patient and family values and preferences.
> - The ethical duty of all healthcare providers includes the obligation to respect diversity in the views of colleagues as well as patients.
> - Interprofessional practice, essential in quality palliative care, requires the support of formal organizational mechanisms such as ethics committees and interdisciplinary rounds

## Overview of Ethical Considerations in Palliative Care

This chapter provides a background and framework for ethical decision making. Basic ethical principles are reviewed, and what Bishop and Scudder refer to as the "primary sense of nursing practice," the moral sense, is addressed.[1] The focus is on the most common issues faced by nurses in palliative care. Goal setting and advanced care planning, resuscitation, proxy decision making, competency and capacity, artificial hydration and nutrition, hastening death, cardiac assistive devices, palliative sedation, and nursing issues such as moral distress and compassion fatigue are some of the topics that are discussed in terms of an ethical framework. The objective of this chapter is to prepare the nurse for identifying and addressing the complex questions that arise in caring for individuals and families facing life-limiting illnesses.

# Ethics and Moral Reasoning

## Definitions

*Ethics,* broadly defined, is the branch of philosophy that is concerned with the study of human conduct, with the rational analysis of how human beings ought to behave and the methods by which we can identify good and evil, right and wrong.[2] In contrast, the term *morality* is conventionally used to refer to accepted and rational codes of conduct governing behavior, aimed to promote good and minimize evil.[3] These terms are closely related and are often used interchangeably.

Given the complexity of the healthcare system and individual patient situations, nurses often are uncertain about the right or most ethically sound action. Moral uncertainty can produce discomfort, but it is the hallmark of a morally sensitive agent. It signals doubt or confusion about values or rules but can usually be resolved with careful analysis.

## In Contrast to Uncertainty

Moral dilemmas are more troublesome and occur when the nurse finds herself or himself in a situation with conflicting demands or one in which every possible action seems to involve violating an ethical duty. Dilemmas may be associated with significant stress and anxiety, resolution may require assistance of others to sort through the conflicts involved. Moral distress is the most damaging state and occurs when the nurse perceives a moral duty but is unable, often because of external constraints, to fulfill that duty. Persistent moral distress can lead to disillusionment, moral apathy, and eventual resignation. Dealing with ethical questions before moral distress occurs requires knowledge and skill in ethical reasoning. A review of the major theories that are the basis for the commonly accepted principles of autonomy, beneficence, nonmaleficence follows.

## Moral Reasoning

Ethics as a discipline has its roots in philosophy. There are many ethical theories that have been developed over the years, each with its own justification. The best known of these are consequentialist theories and deontologic theories. *Consequentialist theories* determine the justification for actions by examining consequences. The action that produces the best consequences for the greatest number is the preferred, or "right" action. *Deontologic theories*, in contrast, argue that actions are right or wrong according to their adherence to duties and obligations, not by virtue of the consequences of the actions. Both types of theories generate principles, such as autonomy (the right of self-determination), beneficence (the duty to promote good), and nonmaleficence (the duty to do no harm).

From principles, in turn, more specific moral rules can be derived. For example, the general duty to respect autonomy and the right of self-determination is the basis of the specific rule that we obtain informed consent before interventions. Both deontologic and consequentialist theories are forms of a "principlist" approach to ethics.

Principlist approaches, although they may rest on differing theoretical premises, all use general and relatively universal principles as the central tool for ethical analysis. Universal principles play a key role in developing mature ethical agency, provide reliable rules of thumb for responding quickly in real-life dilemmas, and reflect the considered wisdom of decades of philosophical analysis. Nevertheless, abstract and somewhat rigid principles can be insensitive to the nuances of specific clinical situations and conflict with deep intuitions of experienced clinicians. Appreciation for the importance of context has grown.

### Feminist Ethics, an Ethic of Care, and Narrative Ethics

Feminist ethics, an outgrowth of the feminist movement, was encouraged by the work of Carol Gilligan, who studied moral reasoning in children and found that boys relied on a rule-oriented, justice-based approach, while girls tended to analyze situations in terms of relationships and context, seeking resolution in the details of the story or narrative.[4]

Consistent with Gilligan's work, caring as a basis for ethics rests on the assumption that morality is rooted in human relationships and feelings. Nel Nodding, recognized as the originator of this theory, argues that morality must stem from the caring instinct and that the ethical ideal is located in the reciprocal caring relationship between and among persons.[5]

Narrative ethics uses the stories of patients and health professionals as the unit of analysis. In seeking understanding of ethical dilemmas from a narrative perspective, the elements of the situation are viewed as components of the story, and aspects such as the relation among participants, predominant voices, intentions of the actors, and consideration of whose voices are heard and not heard are central to developing understanding of the ethical dimensions.[6]

As with the ethic of care and feminist ethics, understanding the relationships among all participants, the meaning of what is stated and unstated, and the motives of all involved is key to the evaluation of how best to respond in ethical dilemmas. Sara Fry has argued that the traditional approach to medical ethics, which centers on application of objective principles and simply evaluating which principle takes priority, is no longer adequate as a foundation for nursing ethics.[7] Fry suggests that nursing ethics rests on a moral view of persons.

The nurse who identifies ethical issues or questions will need to use a systematic process to examine the situation and reach a decision about what action to take. There are many suggested models for analyzing ethical dilemmas, and any thoughtful, deliberative process can be helpful.

One approach that is similar to the problem solving steps most nurses have learned is illustrated in Box 1.1.

## The Process

The process begins with identifying the issue or question; this step helps to focus the ethical issue, clarify what aspect of a complex patient care situation is raising concerns. and differentiate the ethical dilemma from clinical problems.

> **Box 1.1 Steps of Ethical Problem Solving**
>
> 1. Define the problem
>    - Differentiate clinical problems, such as uncertainty or disagreement about prognosis, from ethical problems, such as determining how to balance duties to provide benefit and duties to respect autonomy; ensure that everyone identifies the same issue.
> 2. Clarify facts and assumptions.
>    - Differentiate known facts from assumptions about the situation, such as presumed motives of family members; ensure that all parties have access to the same facts.
> 3. Develop list of all options.
>    - Avoid collapsing options into "yes/no" absolutes, such as "continue all treatment" and "discontinue all treatment"; ensure that all possible actions are evaluated, including intermediate steps such as continue all treatments and escalate as needed; continue all treatments but do not add anything further; discontinue ineffective interventions but continue noninvasive treatments; discontinue all interventions that do not promote comfort.
> 4. Evaluate all options.
>    - Consider relevant laws, policies, and ethical principles; address rights, duties, and interests of all involved.
> 5. Choose the optimal option and implement.

The second step, reviewing facts and assumptions, directs the nurse to be clear about relevant data and sensitive to assumptions that may not be based on adequate data. The third step, listing all options, is intended to prompt the nurse to think carefully about all possible actions, rather than falling into the temptation to dichotomize the possible answers (e.g., withdrawing all treatment or continuing all treatment, accepting the patient's decision or not accepting it).

The fourth step is the point at which the nurse must bring to bear considerations related to ethical principles, relevant professional norms, laws, policies, and personal values. In this step, each option is evaluated against these touchstones or criteria. Then, having evaluated each option, the final decision is made as the fifth step. Most ethical dilemmas are multifaceted with conflicting demands. The need to address them in a methodic and logical process is part of the essential caring role of the nurse in responding to such dilemmas.

### Common Ethical Dilemmas

## Case Study 1: Deciding Whether to Place a Feeding Tube

An 82-year-old man with a 15-year history of coronary artery disease, myocardial infarction, and heart failure enters the hospital with a left-sided cerebrovascular accident (CVA) that has left him partially aphasic and hemiparetic, causing him to aspirate food of any consistency. Seven days after the stroke, his mental status is unclear, and there is disagreement as to whether he has decisional capacity. He is able to answer "yes" and "no," although the responses are inconsistent. The attending physician is convinced that the patient lacks decision-making capacity, but two family members (his wife and older brother) are equally convinced that he has decisional capacity. The patient does not have an advance directive. The patient's wife states that they have never held specific or detailed conversations about preferences for life-sustaining treatment. Until his stroke, he was active in his retirement and enjoyed gardening and playing bridge with friends. She believes he would not want to live in a condition that would not allow him to function as fully as he was before the CVA but is ambivalent about the placement of a feeding tube. The patient's two daughters insist that a feeding tube should be placed because not doing so would be "killing him." The attending physician and the rest of the interdisciplinary healthcare team are opposed to placing the feeding tube. In fact, several nurses who have cared for this patient during previous hospitalizations for heart failure claim that the patient told them that he would not want to be sustained by artificial means. The attending physician, as well as the neurologic consultant, has verified that, at this point, further significant recovery is likely to be minimal because of dense damage to the cerebral cortex. They believe placing a feeding tube would be "futile." The advanced practice nurse is not comfortable with claiming the feeding tube would be "futile" but is concerned about whether the patient would have wanted it and whether it will serve his best interests in the long term. She wonders how to get help in resolving the conflict.

### Goal Setting and Advance Care Planning

Patients with advanced disease or near the end of life, their families, and healthcare providers may encounter a variety of ethical dilemmas and subsequent choices. Although moral questions can arise about any aspect of nursing practice, including informed consent and duties to colleagues, the issues most frequently encountered in palliative care center around end-of-life decisions. These include withholding or withdrawing treatment (e.g., mechanical ventilation, hemodialysis, cardiopulmonary resuscitation, and cardiac assist devices), concerns about use of ANH, requests for hastened death (assisted suicide and euthanasia), and palliative sedation. As a consequence, it is usually more helpful to focus on patient preferences for *outcomes* of treatments rather than preferences or choices for *specific treatments*.[8]

For the most part, ethical analyses of these issues are grounded in patient choices, goals of care, preferences, prognosis, and communication. However, there are many important social, professional, and legal influences that have made these choices complex. The continual expansion of technologic options and biomedical interventions, particularly over the past few decades, has enabled the medical profession to prolong life through sophisticated interventions before adequate bioethical norms have been established. Clearly this requires careful and repeated discussions with patients and their families. As can be seen in Case Study 1, it would have been much more helpful to know the patient's feelings and attitudes about what states or conditions would be acceptable to him rather than general statements about use of "artificial means." The pace and demands of healthcare today add to the challenges of addressing ethical issues in the clinical setting and may lead to hasty and arbitrary decision making. A preventive ethics approach will help ensure that decisions made are thoughtful and beneficial to patients and families.

**Preventive Ethics**

*Preventive ethics* can be thought of as standards and norms that, when adhered to, can minimize the frequency with which difficult conflicts and dilemmas occur. The use of advance care planning is an example of a preventive ethics intervention that nurses can implement on an individual level. The Veterans Administration, as part of their integrated ethics program, has adopted a quality improvement approach to systematizing efforts to address quality gaps, such as lack of attention to and support of advance care planning, and nurses can be key agents in such hospital-wide efforts.[9]

Because of the many difficult decisions that will be faced by most people as they age and as they experience serious illnesses, assuring that thoughtful discussions take place before serious illness occurs can be quite helpful in preventing later uncertainties and dilemmas (see Case Study 1).

*Documentation reflecting advance care planning can take many forms.* Advance care planning is a process of communication and documentation to identify patients' preferences about goals of care and to identify an authorized proxy who can provide competent, confident, and informed representation for choices when the patient is unable to express wishes. Advance directives are written instructions to healthcare providers that are established before the need for medical intervention. Advance directives have three major purposes: (1) to provide a mechanism to enable providers to respect patient autonomy in situations in which the patient cannot express his or her wishes, (2) to provide guidance to healthcare professionals and family members regarding how to proceed with decision making about life-sustaining interventions; and (3) to provide immunity for professionals from civil and criminal liabilities when certain stated conditions are met.

A *living will* is one type of advance directive that is often accompanied by a *durable power of attorney for healthcare* (DPAHC) or health-care proxy. Living wills are used to declare wishes to refuse, limit, or withhold life-sustaining treatment under such circumstances that the individual is incapacitated or unable to communicate. The DPAHC authorizes the agent or proxy to make all healthcare decisions, presumably acting as the patient would have. A living will, as the patient's own treatment preference, takes precedence over the DPAHC if there are conflicts. In many states, the living will statute specifies that this document is only in effect when the patient is terminally ill, as determined by the physician, and thus it may not be helpful in situations such as major CVA, persistent vegetative state, coma, or other serious illnesses that are not considered inevitably terminal.

Despite their shortcomings, advance directives are the best instruments we have to ensure that an individual's goals and preferences for care are met.[10] Because predicting and outlining all possible choices regarding healthcare scenarios is difficult, advance directives are rarely defined as precisely as needed especially when a disease progresses and the context of the situation changes.[11] Although it has been more than two decades since the Patient Self-Determination Act (PSDA) was made law in 1990, empirical studies reporting effectiveness of advance directives have yielded disappointing results. Only 25% to 35% of patients have completed these, even among seriously ill populations such as persons with cancer, and when present, they often do not direct care.[12-14]

Advance care planning is an essential process that should begin to take place at the point of diagnosis and be revisited throughout the course of the disease trajectory to ensure that patients' preferences for care are preserved. Other forms of advance directives include out-of-hospital *do-not-attempt-resuscitation* (DNAR) orders, and the *Five Wishes* a detailed guide for discussions of preferences for end-of-life care.[15] The *Five Wishes* document, recognized in 42 states, helps individuals who are seriously ill and unable to speak for themselves express how they want to be treated from a medical, personal, emotional, and spiritual perspective. In addition, this unique document helps patients discuss their wishes with family and the healthcare team.

Healthcare advance directives differ widely in format and content, making the already complex issues that palliative care nurses face even more difficult. Additional barriers exist when patients transfer from one care facility to another and the requirements change or the previously existing document is not incorporated or honored.[16] In addition, some advance directives are not sufficient to direct care in some healthcare institutions until a physician's order is written in the medical record. These barriers have led to an attempt to remedy these problems through the creation of other methods, such as *physician orders for life-sustaining treatment* (POLST) and *medical orders for life-sustaining treatment* (MOLST).[17,18] The overall aim of these newer forms of advance directives is to improve the communication of personal wishes about life-sustaining treatments, resulting in higher quality medical care that is consistent with patient choice.

The *POLST Paradigm* was originally developed in Oregon to improve end-of-life care by overcoming many of the shortcomings and pitfalls of advance directives.[16,19] The POLST document is designed to be long-lasting and portable across treatment settings and can be posted on the patient's refrigerator or on the front of the patient's medical record, where it can be easily located by emergency medical personnel and other healthcare providers.

The cornerstone of the program is a brightly colored, standardized form that provides specific treatment orders for mechanical ventilation, antibiotics, cardiopulmonary resuscitation, and ANH. It is recommended for persons who have a life-limiting disease, who might die in the next year, or who want to further define their preferences for care and treatment.

Other states have adopted similar programs with different names, although all share the same core elements and with similar forms (e.g., POLST in West Virginia; MOLST in New York).[20]

The National Consensus Project for Quality Palliative Care, third edition, of the Clinical Practice Guidelines for Quality Palliative Care[21] recommends that the POLST model be adopted nationwide because it more accurately reflects treatment goals and ensures that the information is transferable and applicable across all healthcare settings.

Although the goals of these newer forms are intended to honor patients' wishes, end-of-life decisions are more nuanced and context dependent than standard "contractual" forms can adequately handle.

*Nursing responsibilities related to advance care planning* include initiating conversations about patient overall goals and specific wishes related to hospitalization, using cardiopulmonary resuscitation and other forms of advanced life support, focusing on values rather than specific treatments, and asking patients and families about the existence of advance directives. Nurses also facilitate access to the documents, teach how to complete them, and help patients and other decision makers think through the patient's wishes. Education about both the formal documents and the process of advance care planning is a critical responsibility in palliative care.

## Do-Not-Attempt-Resuscitation Orders

Decisions about the level and type of interventions to be used must stem from consensus about the goals of care. For patients in acute care settings and those who have not yet elected to focus on comfort rather than cure or life prolongation, the specific issue of resuscitation status is a frequent source of distress for clinicians as well as patients and families. In addition to discomfort and inexperience with the topic, there continues to be widespread misunderstanding about the efficacy of cardiopulmonary resuscitation (CPR) efforts and the meaning of decisions to withhold CPR in the event of an arrest.

### Facts About Cardiopulmonary Resuscitation

In acute care settings, cardiopulmonary resuscitation is successful in supporting survival to hospital discharge in only about 18% of instances of arrest.[22] This success rate has changed little in the 50 years since the technique of CPR was first developed. The relative ineffectiveness of CPR reflects the inappropriate widespread use of resuscitation efforts in situations in which multiple preexisting chronic illnesses have led to an irreversible state and death is inevitable. The public has little understanding of what actually occurs in CPR, the limited benefit except in situations of single-organ disease and immediate intervention, and the potential for cognitive impairment if circulation is restored.[23]

Clinicians may inadvertently contribute to misunderstandings about CPR in several ways, including avoiding discussions of goals of care and raising the topic of resuscitation status in the form of a question to patients or to families, such as "What do you want us to do if his heart stops?" This approach is misguided because it places full responsibility for decision making on the patient or family and implies that CPR has a good chance of being successful.

### DNAR in Place of DNR: The Rationale

The American Heart Association converted to the acronym DNAR (do not attempt resuscitation) from the formerly used DNR (do not resuscitate) in their 2005 standards,[24] for the following reasons:

- It is important to signal recognition that CPR, with its current wide application, more accurately is an *attempt* to restore cardiac function.
- This attempt is most often unsuccessful, and this change in language facilitates recognition that a DNAR order does not entail a decision to allow a preventable death to occur.
- A DNAR order indicates a decision to withhold a very invasive and aggressive intervention that has little chance in promoting survival to hospital discharge.

Clarification of resuscitation status is part of overall care planning. Because CPR in the event of an arrest is the default in virtually all healthcare settings, resuscitation status must be addressed in every situation of life-limiting or serious illness. This is particularly important when patients change care settings or begin care with new providers, such as admission to a long-term care facility, home healthcare, or home hospice. In addition to discussion of overall goals and quality of life, the nurse can provide factual information about CPR and clarify the difference between a plan to withhold this ineffective intervention and the plan to use maximal efforts to prevent cardiac arrest.

Although use of DNAR orders is the standard method to indicate to healthcare personnel that CPR is not to be used, these orders are only effective within the facility in which they are issued. The need to have portable orders and valid indicators of DNAR status for patients moving between facilities or patients being cared for at home has led to the creation of out-of-hospital forms and identifiers. As of 2002, 42 states had passed legislation authorizing statewide "out-of-hospital" DNAR protocols.[25] All nurses have a responsibility to be familiar with their state's forms and protocols to ensure that decisions to forego CPR remain in place as patients transition among care settings.

Unlike most advance directives, the out-of-hospital DNAR document is a valid physician order that takes effect as soon as it is signed; it is not limited by the patient's diagnosis or terminal status. When available, these forms should be initiated when the decision to forego CPR is first made so that patients can take them with them as they are discharged or transferred among facilities.

A frequent challenge nurses face is how to manage situations in which they perceive the patient's condition is deteriorating and no one has addressed the issue of resuscitation status with the patient or family.

Common concerns are that initiating such a discussion is outside the boundaries of the nursing role, that physicians will be angry if the nurse raises the topic, and that patients or families will be upset. Kirchhoff and colleagues reported on the perceptions of obstacles and helpful behaviors that 199 critical care nurses discussed in providing end-of-life care to dying patients.[26] The highest ranked "helpful" was "having all physicians agree about the direction of care." This ranking may reflect the degree of distress nurses feel when "stuck in the middle." It is important for nurses to recognize that it is within the professional role of nursing to identify the need to develop consensus around goals of care and treatment plans and to facilitate discussions surrounding difficult decision making.

## Proxy Decision Making

Because patients with serious illness frequently lack cognitive capacity at some point during the illness, professionals must rely on family or friends to represent their wishes and participate in decision making. This creates a number of possible areas of conflict and uncertainty, including the need to make careful assessments of capacity, questions about the moral authority of family and friends to make decisions for patients, and in some cases, the need to manage conflicts among and between families and the care team, as occurred in Case Study 1.

### Competency and Capacity

*Incompetency* refers to a status that is conferred by a court, establishing the inability of an individual to act as an autonomous and legally responsible person. Only the court can make a determination of *competence*; clinicians provide evidence to the court regarding the *capacity* of the individual, including data about diagnosis, cognitive and functional ability, and likelihood of recovery. An individual who has been deemed "incompetent" loses the right to make all decisions, including healthcare decisions, and must have a guardian appointed by the court to manage all affairs.[27]

Clinicians cannot establish competency but have an ongoing responsibility to assess capacity of the patient to participate in decision making. When patients are not able to express their wishes or make decisions and do not have a designated healthcare agent, family members are asked to act as proxies. Although this is common practice, states vary in the extent to which this is authorized by law and the precise specification of which family members have priority in decision making.

### Justification for Members to Act as Proxies

The moral basis for allowing one adult to make decisions for another is the assumption that family members are committed to furthering the best interests of the patient and family members, who share background, experiences, religion, and culture with the patient and are well equipped to represent the preferences and values of the patient. These assumptions are usually quite valid, but there are situations in which nurses question the ability of the family member to act as a valid proxy for the patient. In these cases, establishing that the assumptions necessary to justify relying on the proxy are, in fact, not confirmed is important in making a plan to seek another representative for that patient. These situations are difficult, and nurses must be prepared to seek guidance from the hospital ethics committee or hospital legal counsel as well as to collaborate with physicians and social workers on the care team. Proxy decision making, even under the best of circumstances, can be very burdensome to families already stressed by the realization of the seriousness of their loved one's illness.

Several studies have demonstrated that family members are not able to consistently identify the preferences of their ill relative even when an advance directive is in place.[28,29] An additional common occurrence is lack of consensus among family members about specific decisions, such as limiting treatment, DNAR status, or referrals to hospice.

In the absence of formal advance directives, intrafamily conflict, as exemplified in Case Study 1, is not uncommon. In that case, the patient's wife seemed to be leaning against use of ANH, but the patient's daughters felt compelled to provide them. Even if the patient had completed a DPAHC that established the wife's authority as a decision maker, the nurse could have provided significant assistance to the family, as a unit, through education, as discussed in the next section, and helping the family come to consensus.

The following is a list of steps the nurse can take to prevent or minimize concerns related to proxy decision making, particularly when initiating palliative care services:

1. All patients who have a serious illness and do not have a DPAHC should be asked to identify a proxy to make decisions if they should become unable. This can be done on admission to the hospital or any other healthcare delivery system in a non-threatening manner, simply pointing out that sometimes patients become too ill or too sleepy because of medication to make decisions for themselves. This enables the team to know, if there are disagreements later, who has the strongest claim to the decision-maker role.

2. The time to obtain information about the patient's lifestyle, values, and preferences is *before* specific decisions about pursuing invasive diagnostic tests or procedures are needed. Talking with family members about what the patient was like, enjoyed, and found important can be helpful in later discussions.

3. When it is necessary to ask a family proxy to provide input into the plan of care, it is essential to address the task as one of helping the clinicians to know what the patient would have wanted. This can be done by referring back to earlier discussions about what was most important to the patient. The goals here are twofold:
    a. To minimize the burden of responsibility the family member might feel
    b. To remain focused on the ethical mandate to act according to the patient's wishes, not the family members' wishes.

Table 1.1 provides examples of ways to phrase questions that are not helpful and of ways that can be more useful in supporting family decision making. In addition, a number of more detailed communication suggestions have been published.[8]

Table 1.1 Phrases to Avoid and Phrases That Can Be More Helpful

| Do Not Say | Do Say |
|---|---|
| "What do you want us to do if your loved one's heart stops?" | "We need to talk about where we go from here if your loved one's condition continues to worsen." |
| "Would you want us to do CPR if your loved one's heart stops?" | "There are many things we can do, but it's very important that we talk together about what your loved one would want done in this situation. Have you and he/she ever known anyone who was this ill? Did he/she say anything about what he/she would want in a situation like this?" |
| "We need your permission to do a (tracheostomy, PEG, angiogram, etc.)" | "Given what we've discussed about your loved one's situation and the most likely benefits and burdens of the procedure, we need your help to know if he/she would want us to proceed with the (tracheostomy, PEG, angiogram, etc.)" |
| "We'll do whatever youw want us to ... it's your decision ... we'll support whatever you decide" | "We have to make some decisions about where to go from here. It's our job to give you information about the medical facts and our recommendations, and we need you to help us know what would be important to your loved one now. Then, we need to talk and come up with a plan together." |

## Artificial Hydration and Nutrition

A fundamental care-giving task is to provide food and fluids. The provision of nutrition and hydration symbolizes the essence of care and compassion, and eating serves as a symbol of health. In most societies, celebrations involve eating, and through these traditional social events we communicate sharing and well-being. Clearly, human life is represented as social and communal through the provision of food.[30]

When a loved one has an advanced illness, these opportunities wane, and when one is dying, they are often lost. However, providing ANH is not synonymous with eating or feeding another person. In health, people eat in a socially acceptable form, with others, in a social setting. Medically provided nutrition and hydration do not share these social characteristics.

The technology of feeding tubes was developed to address specific temporary medical problems (e.g., postsurgical gastric motility issues, swallowing impairment following a stroke in a patient expected to recover). However, feeding tubes and medically provided nutrition and hydration have become widely used in patients with very poor prognoses and in those with little likelihood of regaining functional abilities. Few decisions are more value laden than those to withhold or withdraw a medical intervention that is thought to be able to prolong life.

As with all decisions about the use of any medical device or treatment, this decision should be based on the patient's goals of care, the medical need, and the burdens and benefits of the treatment. In general, patients (or their surrogates) have the right to withhold or withdraw ANH if they believe that the burden or risks outweigh the benefits. There is widespread agreement in ethics and law[31-33] that patients or their surrogates have a right to choose or refuse ANH. All decisions about nutrition and hydration should be made in light of patient's goals and outcomes of care. These goals of care may change during the course of the disease or as the disease progresses and the patient's cognitive and physical functioning decline. Consequently, nurses should create opportunities for discussion and negotiation of goals and priorities of care with the patient and family or surrogate on an ongoing basis.

ANH require the placement of a temporary or permanent feeding tube or the initiation of intravenous access. These interventions are associated with risks, including the following:

- Bleeding, tube displacement, and infection, as well as the potential need for repositioning and replacement,[34,35]
- In patients with impaired renal function, intravenous fluids may promote peripheral or pulmonary edema and increase the need for suctioning.[36]
- Other potential side effects of tube feeding include diarrhea, nausea, vomiting, and aspiration of the feeding into the lung.[36] Tube feedings do not appear to prevent aspiration pneumonia and may increase the risk compared with that in patients who do not take anything by mouth.[34]

Empirical data by Teno and colleagues[37] concluded that feeding tubes are not associated with prevention or improved healing of a pressure ulcer.[37] Hospitalized nursing home residents who received a percutaneous endoscopic gastrostomy (PEG) tube were 2.7 times more likely to develop a new pressure ulcer, and those with a pressure ulcer were less likely to show healing of the ulcer when they had a PEG inserted. Similarly, there is particularly strong evidence confirming the failure of PEGs and tube feeding to prolong survival in states of advanced dementia.[34,35,38,39]

## Addressing Family Concerns

Many patients and family members have deep concerns about the issues of "hunger" and "starvation." Contrary to what many believe, a patient with a terminal disease, who is often anorexic from the effects of the disease, may not be bothered by hunger.[40] Additionally, many patients in whom the disease is progressing report a complete lack of hunger. Evidence suggests that natural physiologic processes that accompany the cessation of food and fluid intake naturally suppress both hunger and thirst. There is strong consensus among palliative care clinicians and oncology professionals that use of parenteral hydration in terminally ill patients is most often associated with unpleasant symptoms of fluid retention and overload.[41]

Nursing interventions that can assist with the palliation of symptoms associated with dry mouth or thirst include small sips of oral intake, ice chips, meticulous mouth care, and lubrication of the lips. Involving caregivers, family members, and loved ones in this activity may replace the family's desire and need to feed with another caregiving activity that can provide the family with the opportunity to provide physical comfort.

### Financial Implications

Some hospice programs cover the cost of ANH, based on the individual plan of care and the goals of care, but others do not. Some extended-care facilities (i.e., nursing homes) mandate medically provided nutrition and hydration when a person stops eating or drinking, often related to misunderstanding and concern about state regulations or related to philosophy and religious missions. Discussions with families about decisions to use ANH, as in Case Study 1, should include consideration of these factors. In Case Study 1, the nurse would have several responsibilities, including clarifying the facts about the patient's previously stated wishes, educating all family members regarding the likely benefits and burdens of tube feedings, and focusing discussions with both physicians and family members on what was known about the patient's values and preferences.

Despite the lack of proven benefit in states of irreversible and advanced illness, ANH will remain an emotionally laden topic and one of the most difficult decisions. Nurses have a particularly important role in educating patients, families, and other members of the healthcare team about the benefits and burdens of tube feedings. There is a persistent widespread belief, particularly among unlicensed assistive personnel and even among some physicians,[42] that we have a duty to feed all patients and that the benefits of ANH always outweigh the burdens. This misunderstanding, in combination with concerns about causing suffering, is a significant barrier to careful ethical evaluation of the decision to use or withhold ANH. Assuring informed decision making about this aspect of the care plan often must begin with addressing the concerns of the care team before developing a plan to make clear recommendations to families and providing family members with the necessary education about this issue.

## Case Study 2: Withdrawal of Life Support in the Intensive Care Unit

Ms. H was a 32-year-old white woman. She was divorced from her husband and had custody of her son, age 6 years, and her daughter, age 3 years. Her parents and her fiancé were her significant others. Ms. H was diagnosed with a uterine leiomyosarcoma 2 years ago. She had undergone two regimens of chemotherapy following a hysterectomy, but the cancer had metastasized to her hip and her mediastinum. The thoracic lesion had grown to the point at which it was compressing her bronchus, and she was taken to the surgery department for stint placement as a palliative measure. This could not be done, and she was then admitted to the intensive care unit, intubated, and placed on mechanical ventilation. Over the course of a week, several attempts were made to extubate her, but she was unable to maintain a patent airway without the positive pressure of the ventilator and the endotracheal tube. Each time the ventilator support was reduced, Ms. H became very anxious and short of breath, even with the use of increasing doses of lorazepam and morphine. She was awake and alert and able to write notes.

On rounds, the ICU attending physician mentioned to the team that it was time to think about doing a tracheostomy because it looked as if Ms. H was not able to be extubated. Ms. P, her nurse, was concerned that this would just subject Ms. H to another procedure and would not change the eventual outcome. She also was uncertain whether anyone had told Ms. H the details of her condition and the real possibility that she would never be able to leave the ICU. On the other hand, the fact that Ms. H was wide awake made it seem as if withdrawing life support (e.g., extubating her) might be cruel—how could this be done without causing suffering?

## Hastening Death—Making Distinctions

A central issue in decision making in states of serious illness is the moral acceptability of actions that can be seen as hastening death. It is well established in Western bioethics that competent patients have an almost unlimited right to accept or refuse medical interventions, regardless of the established efficacy of the intervention or its necessity for survival. Supporting and advocating for this right is a critical function of the nurse and one that has been identified as a frequent source of ethical distress.

The recognized right of the individual to elect to stop life-sustaining technology, such as mechanical ventilation or hemodialysis, has been used by some as the basis for arguing that there is no difference between this act and acts that intentionally hasten death, including both euthanasia and assisted suicide. Arguments that there is a difference usually rely on the distinction between allowing a death caused by disease, as occurs when removing unwanted or ineffective life-prolonging therapies such as mechanical ventilators and dialysis, and killing, which entails being the direct cause of death (see Case Studies 1 and 2). Each nurse who cares for patients with life-limiting disease will have to carefully identify his or her own beliefs regarding discontinuing life-prolonging therapy.

### Definitions—Distinction Between Euthanasia and Assisted Suicide

*Euthanasia* is defined as an intentional act performed for the purpose of causing the death of another for reasons of mercy. Euthanasia in all forms is illegal in the United States and is condoned by none of the professional associations (Box 1.2). *Assisted suicide* is the provision of assistance in some form (e.g., supplying lethal medications or instructions) to an individual who then acts to take his or her own life. Assisted suicide (also termed physician-aid-in-dying and physician-assisted suicide [PAS]) has been legal in Oregon since 1997 and was most recently approved by voters in Washington State.[43] At this time, professional nursing organizations do not condone nurses actively participating in assisted suicide.

Nurses, as the healthcare professionals who spend the greatest amount of time with patients and their families and who often have the most intimate relationships with them, are inevitably involved in situations involving the issue of hastening death. This may take the form of explicit requests

## Box 1.2 Position Statements From Recognized Professional Organizations

### Artificial Hydration and Nutrition

Hospice and Palliative Nurses Association (HPNA). *Position Statement—Artificial Nutrition and Hydration in Advanced Illness.* Pittsburgh, PA: Hospice and Palliative Nurses Association; 2011.

National Hospice and Palliative Care Organization (NHPCO). *Position Statement—Artificial Nutrition and Hydration Narrative and Statement.* Alexandria, VA: National Hospice and Palliative Care Organization; 2010.

American Nurses Association (ANA). *Position Statement—Foregoing Nutrition and Hydration.* Washington, DC: American Nurses Association; 2011.

American Academy of Hospice and Palliative Medicine (AAHPM). *Position Statement—Artificial Nutrition and Hydration Near the End of Life.* Glenview, IL: American Academy of Hospice and Palliative Medicine; 2006.

### Physician-Assisted Suicide

Hospice and Palliative Nurses Association (HPNA). *Position Statement—Legalization of Assisted Suicide.* Pittsburgh, PA: Hospice and Palliative Nurses Association; 2011.

National Hospice and Palliative Care Organization (NHPCO). *Commentary and Resolution—Physician Assisted Suicide.* Alexandria, VA: National Hospice and Palliative Care Organization; 2010.

American Academy of Hospice and Palliative Medicine (AAHPM). *Position Statement—Physician Assisted Death.* Glenview, IL: American Academy of Hospice and Palliative Medicine; 2007.

Oncology Nursing Society. *Nurse's Responsibility to the Patient Requesting Assistance in Hastening Death.* Pittsburgh, PA: Oncology Nursing Society; 2010.

American Society for Pain Management Nursing. *Position Statement—Assisted Suicide.* Lenexa, KS: American Society for Pain Management Nursing; 2011.

### Palliative Sedation

Hospice and Palliative Nurses Association (HPNA). *Position Statement—Palliative Sedation.* Pittsburgh, PA: Hospice and Palliative Nurses Association; 2011.

American Academy of Hospice and Palliative Medicine (AAHPM). *Position Statement—Palliative Sedation.* Glenview, IL: American Academy of Hospice and Palliative Medicine; 2006.

National Hospice and Palliative Care Organization. *Position Statement—Use of Palliative Sedation in Imminently Dying Terminally Ill Patients.* Alexandria, VA: National Hospice and Palliative Care Organization; 2010.

National Hospice and Palliative Care Organization. *Position Statement—Palliative Sedation in Hospice and Palliative Care.* Alexandria, VA: National Hospice and Palliative Care Organization; 2012.

from patients for some action that would precipitate death or shorten survival. Patients and families may request information or counseling from the nurse regarding hastening death, or nurses may identify more subtle clues that the patient or family are considering hastening death. The desire for hastened death at some point in terminal illness has been found to occur with relative frequency. Emanuel and colleagues[44] reported an incidence of serious consideration for either euthanasia or PAS in 10.6% of 988 terminally ill patients. O'Mahony and associates[45] found that 34% of 131 patients admitted to a palliative care service had some level of desire for hastening death. In a large Dutch survey of nurses' involvement in end-of-life decisions in hospitals, nursing homes, and home care, the nurse was the first person with whom the patient discussed a request for euthanasia or PAS in 45.1% of cases.[46] These situations require very careful attention from the nurse, awareness of legal and ethical considerations, and a well-developed and collaborative plan for responding.

Nursing responsibilities when a patient expresses thoughts of a hastened death are clarification and assessment. The expression of thoughts of hastening death may be an accurate report of a serious intention, a relatively off-hand comment, an expression of distress prompted by unrelieved symptoms, or intended as a test of the nurse's views about hastening death. A thorough evaluation of the adequacy of symptom management, particularly pain and depression, is necessary. Ganzini and associates found that among 58 patients in Oregon who sought PAS, 26% were assessed as depressed on psychiatric interview.[47]

A number of guidelines have been developed by professional associations and groups to assist the clinician in responding to requests for hastened death.[48,49] All of these emphasize the right of professionals to withdraw from situations in which they are being requested to act in a way, such as participating in assisted suicide, that violates their moral principles. Professionals have an absolute duty, however, to assure patients that they will not be abandoned, to work diligently to investigate and address correctable factors that may be leading to the request for hastened death, and to refrain from withdrawing until an alternate source of care is in place.

## Special Questions: Cardiac Assist Devices, Palliative Sedation, and Medical Futility

Three specific issues present particularly challenging questions in palliative care: (1) the acceptability and methods of withdrawing life-sustaining interventions that consist of cardiac assistive devices (pacemakers, automatic internal cardiodefibrillators [AICDs], left ventricular assistive devices [LVADs]); (2) concerns about requests for futile therapy; and (3) palliative sedation.

### Cardiac Assistive Devices

One of the most concrete examples of the complexities created by advancing technologies is the situation of patients who have elected to forego continued use of cardioassistive devices to allow a peaceful death. There are a number of implantable mechanical assistive devices intended to either support or replace normal cardiac electrical and mechanical function, including

LVADs, right ventricular assistive devices (RVADs), total implantable hearts (TIHs), internal AICDs, and pacemakers. Each of these raises unique issues.

Internal AICDs are commonly used in the United States in the treatment of recurrent ventricular fibrillation. Pacemakers have been a long-standing therapy for bradyarrhythmias, and combined AICD-pacemakers are recommended for some forms of heart failure.

In an international survey in 2005, 223,425 pacemakers and 119,121 AICDs were implanted in the United States.[50] It is therefore very likely that palliative care nurses will find themselves caring for patients with either or both of these devices. In most cases, both AICDs and pacemakers are on-demand therapy; that is, they are programmed to deliver therapy only on demand (when heart rate decreases or a lethal arrhythmia develops). Their function should be disabled when the plan of care is based on a goal of allowing a peaceful death with no further intervention. AICDs should be turned off so that they will not deliver a shock as the heart rate falls or ventricular arrhythmias occur. Demand pacemakers can have the rate and sensitivity decreased so that they do not prolong the dying process. Cardiologists or cardiac technicians usually must be called and requested to make these changes using the device programming magnets.

When cardiac function is dependent on active device operation, as is the case with some pacemakers and most cardiac-assistive devices, there are more difficult challenges and unresolved questions. Some argue that discontinuing a cardiac assist device, with the expectation that death will follow, is no different, morally, than discontinuing mechanical ventilation for a patient who has elected (or whose family has elected) to have life-sustaining therapy discontinued.

Others believe that the fact that the device is implanted and has become, in a sense, part of the patient makes discontinuation equivalent to an act of euthanasia and thus is impermissible.[51-53]

Since 2002, LVADs have been considered "destination therapy" for patients who are ineligible for transplantation or whose estimated 1-year mortality is greater than 50% with medical therapy.[54] LVADs will alter end-of-life trajectories. Although intended to prolong survival related to heart failure, LVADs have the potential to decrease the overall quality of life of these patients because of serious infections, neurologic complications, and device malfunction.[55-57]

Numerous nurse-led research studies have shed light on the importance of the ethical obligations nurses hold to provide significant emotional support to these patients and their families.[58,59] When caring for the patient with an implanted cardiac device, the nurse has several responsibilities. The exact status of the device's operation has to be determined. The plan for adjusting the device should stem from a clear understanding of the patient's goals of care. If the goal is to make the most of whatever time is left and there is hope for more time, all cardiac devices should remain active and in place. If the patient is actively dying or has expressed an informed desire to remove any therapy that could interfere with the dying process (whenever that might occur), the devices should be inactivated (or turned to an inactive setting).

Each of these decisions must be made in collaboration with the care team. If there is consensus about discontinuing a device on which cardiac function is entirely dependent, extra care must be taken to ensure that the patient, family members, and entire care team are in agreement. Although, as with ANH, there is still some lack of consensus among healthcare professionals about the morality of discontinuing cardiac assist devices, there is formal agreement from the relevant medical professional organization (Heart Rhythm Society) that discontinuing this form of therapy is no different than the withdrawal of any other form of unwanted or ineffective therapy.[60] The timing of the discontinuation must be carefully considered and a plan to address likely symptoms put in place.

*Palliative Sedation*
There are few situations at the end of life in which patient symptoms cannot be adequately relieved despite multiple pharmacologic regimens. Even with the provision of evidence-based, state-of-the-art palliative care, some patients will continue to experience protracted, intense suffering toward the end of life. In these cases, the option of palliative sedation is sometimes raised. *Palliative sedation* refers to the use of medications to induce sedation, either intermittently or continuously, for the purpose of providing relief of intractable symptoms. The intention is not to cause death. In an effort to clarify the different types of palliative sedation and how each may be used, Quill and colleagues[61] outlined three kinds of sedation: ordinary, proportionate, and palliative sedation to unconsciousness.

If the goal of care is to relieve the symptoms without reduction of level of consciousness, *ordinary sedation* could serve as a treatment intervention.

With *proportionate palliative sedation* (PPS), pharmaceutical agents such as benzodiazepines are progressively escalated to induce increasing levels of sedation during both waking and sleeping hours. This type of sedation is usually employed for intractable physical suffering in imminently dying patients.

If unconsciousness is the intended goal of care rather than a side effect, *palliative sedation to unconsciousness* (PSU) can be used.

## Concern That Palliative Sedation Hastens Death

Although these definitions have helped to clarify the types of sedation, there remains concern that access to these practices may become too easy. In a recent systematic review of the literature regarding palliative sedation and survival, Maltoni and colleagues[62] found no evidence to suggest that palliative sedation has any detrimental effect on survival of patients with terminal cancer. They suggest that it is a medical intervention that should be included in the repertoire of interventions to relieve suffering.

Wide variation in the use of palliative sedation and limited research about best practice may reflect ambivalence and uncertainty about the ethical acceptability of the practice.[63]

The most common objection to palliative sedation is the belief that PPS and PSU will directly hasten death. A review of published data by Claessens and colleagues[64] indicates that this is not the case. Use of PPS and PSU require addressing other interventions, such as the continuation of oral medications and the administration of food and fluids. In general, these other decisions should be made separately and before palliative sedation is begun. If there are adequate reasons to stop food, fluids, and other medications (i.e., if the patient is in the final stages of dying, has been refusing food and fluids, and other medications are not needed for promotion of comfort), there is no reason to insist they be used when palliative sedation begins. If nutrition and hydration were indicated before sedation, there may be good reason to continue their use, or sedation should be stopped or lightened intermittently to offer food and fluid.

Case Study 2 is an example of a situation in which palliative sedation might be necessary. If Ms. H, who retained decisional capacity, chose to have ventilator support withdrawn, it might be necessary to sedate her to the point of unconsciousness to prevent suffering. The act of discontinuing ventilator support would in all probability shorten her survival compared with continuing mechanical ventilation. However, this act would be morally permissible and supported by the principle of double effect.

## The Principle of Double Effect

Well established in bioethics, the *principle of double effect* asserts that acts that are intended to achieve a "good" effect (in this case, respecting autonomy and preventing suffering) are permissible even if the act also carries with it an unintended "bad" effect (hastened death). The principle requires that the good not be achieved by means of the bad (i.e., the relief of suffering is achieved by the sedation, not by causing death) and that the weight of the good achieved must be greater than the bad effect.[30]

Although the American Academy of Hospice and Palliative Medicine, the National Hospice and Palliative Care Organization, and the Hospice and Palliative Nurses Association (see Box 1.2) support the use of palliative sedation in carefully selected situations, all organizations emphasize the importance of clarity in the intended objective (relief of suffering) and the need for thorough discussion and informed consent from the patient. In addition, all organizations providing palliative and end-of-life care should have a written policy or guidelines about palliative sedation and the types of sedation that will be offered to patients if requested. This policy should be provided to patients or their proxies who ask about the possibility of having PSU in the future or request it when other interventions have failed to relieve intractable suffering. Moreover, if the organization offers PSU but an individual physician objects to its provision, the organization or clinician must make alternative arrangements for the care to be transferred to another provider or institution. Given the importance of communication in the final stages of life, use of palliative sedation should be reserved for those few situations in which all other interventions have been ineffective and the patient finds continued consciousness to be intolerable.

## Futility

*Futility* is a term that refers to the inability of a specific intervention to lead to its intended outcome (e.g., prolonged survival, discharge from the hospital, shrinkage of tumor). This term has gained popularity in acute care over the past decade as clinicians have increasingly encountered situations in which patients and families request or demand therapies that the clinician believes have no meaningful chance of prolonging life or improving well-being.[65-67] There is growing consensus that the right of patients and families to accept or refuse therapies does not entail the right to demand therapies that the physician does not believe are medically justified.[68] The right to accept or refuse therapy stems from the principle of autonomy. This principle establishes the duty to refrain from interfering in the life choices of competent persons; it is thus a "liberty right," not a right to demand access to any particular intervention.

The move away from the paternalism and a commitment to supporting patient autonomy has led to a tendency to shift the responsibility for decision making entirely to patients and families. This is sometimes seen in the reluctance of clinicians to advise or guide patients and families in decisions and, instead, to present options in a completely impartial fashion. Clinicians then may find themselves facing situations in which patients or families demand therapies that are thought to offer little benefit and significant probability of harm. Most often, this occurs with the question of resuscitation status or continued use of chemotherapy in advanced refractory cancer.[69,70] The frequency of futility dilemmas and the difficulty in resolving them has led professional organizations and many other healthcare organizations to develop policies for managing conflict. Although these policies are important in providing general guidelines for physicians and nurses, it is far more important to attempt to prevent futility conflicts from developing. As with most ethical dilemmas, effective communication and trusting relationships are key.

*Steps nurses can take to lessen the likelihood of development of irreconcilable differences* include the following:

1. Begin with talking early about goals of care, learning about the values and beliefs of the patient and family, and establishing a collaborative model of decision making. Not infrequently, families will express the wish to have "everything" done for their loved one. When this is said, the nurse or physician should respond by assuring the patient and family that they are heard and that their wish to receive all therapies that have any meaningful chance of maintaining or improving the patient's condition will be used. The use of shared decision making should be emphasized from the start.

2. As the condition of the patient deteriorates and it becomes apparent that continued interventions will not be helpful, it is best to set the stage for later decisions by affirming that the clinicians will provide honest and direct information and will identify when there are no further curative options, with assurances that the plan of care will always be discussed before changes are made.

3. When the situation is such that CPR or other interventions are no longer indicated, this should be stated; patients or families should not be asked to give permission to withhold an ineffective intervention.

4. If consensus appears to be unreachable, other resources, such as clergy or ethics consultants, should be used. Although seeking guidance from

the court may be required in intractable disputes, in general this should be viewed as a last resort, and thoughtful, interdisciplinary procedural approaches are preferable.[71,72]

In Case Study 2, the nurse, Ms. P, may have believed that performing a tracheostomy on Ms. H would indeed be futile. Although the procedure could be safely performed, it would not save the patient's life or even allow her to recover enough to leave the ICU—she would always require mechanical ventilation. To address this issue, Ms. P would need to validate her assumption about the location of Ms. H's tumor and the ineffectiveness of a tracheostomy to relieve the obstruction and arrange for a care conference with the entire multidisciplinary team to arrive at consensus about the best approach. If the team reached agreement about the lack of any effective treatment options for the cancer, a plan would have to be developed, including who would talk with Ms. H, what recommendation would be offered, what options would be acceptable, and how her symptoms would be managed when she was ready to discontinue mechanical ventilation.

Although it is recognized that clinicians have not only the right but also the professional duty to refrain from interventions that are harmful, it is essential to be cautious in judging interventions as futile. There are many treatments or therapies that offer neither cure nor improvement in patient condition but are effective in supporting survival, such as mechanical ventilation following anoxic brain injuries. The claim of futility should not be used to justify withholding therapies in situations in which the clinician believes that the proposed therapy would accomplish its intended purpose but the resulting quality of life would be undesirable. Judgments such as this reflect the subjective opinions and values of clinicians and are not a valid basis for withholding therapy against the wishes of patients and families.

## Nursing Issues, Moral Distress, and Compassion Fatigue

With increased medical technology, the advances in science, and conflicting interests of patients and families, nurses stand in a pivotal position to lead the way in ensuring patient access to quality palliative care. This charge does not come without the risk of the nurse being put "in the middle," trying to provide the best possible care to the patient and supporting the family members while bracketing personal values.[73]

Nurses and other members of the interdisciplinary healthcare team face ethical and legal issues in decision making related to end-of-life care daily in clinical practice. These dilemmas have a strong potential to provoke conflict among those involved in patient care, sometimes between professionals and sometimes between patients, families, and professionals. The American Nurses Association (ANA) Code of Ethics for Nurses states that nurses have the right to withdraw from providing care to patients when their own values conflict with that of patient, as long as the patient's care can safely be transferred to another care provider.

Caring for patients with advanced illness brings with it complex clinical situations and ethical challenges; nurses must find ways to support one another through talking and sharing experiences about moral uncertainty. The Code of Ethics for Nurses urges nurses to collaborate with colleagues to advocate for healthcare environments conducive to ethical practice and to the health and well-being of all in the setting and to do so in ways consistent with professional behavior. The ANA goes on to discuss the importance of "preservation of integrity." Specifically, provisions 5 and 6 of the ANA Code of Ethics discuss moral self-respect and the influence of the environment on ethical obligations, moral virtues, and values. According to these provisions, nurses have a duty to remain consistent with both their personal and professional values and to possess character strengths such as compassion and patience. Although simply stated, these behaviors may become challenged when faced with ethical and moral dilemmas.

Nurses, like other licensed professionals, profess to society that they are prepared to take on certain responsibilities in safe, competent, and ethical ways. Many nurses enter the profession by taking a pledge, such as the Florence Nightingale Pledge, swearing to devote themselves to others who require their care, knowledge, and expertise. Every day, hospice and palliative care nurses provide care to patients who rely on them for not only physical care needs but also psychological, social, and spiritual care. Close, personal relationships are often formed with patients and their family as palliative care nurses care for them over a prolonged period of time. In a large survey of nurses from a variety of healthcare settings, including hospice, ICU, nursing facilities, and inpatient care, Ferrell[74] identified that nurses' greatest sources of moral distress originated from "aggressive care" and "aggressive care denying palliative care." Moral and ethical dilemmas, often associated with patient and family situations, and healthcare environments may leave the hospice and palliative care nurse feeling physically, emotionally, and spiritually drained. As nurses continue to be exposed to patients with greater healthcare needs, staff shortages, heavy and intense workloads, an aging workforce, and a lack of resources to work effectively, the opportunity to develop moral distress, moral fatigue, burnout, and compassion fatigue is glaring.

### Compassion Fatigue

*Compassion fatigue* is a relatively new term yet is pervasive within the nursing profession.[75] Compassion fatigue is a state in which the compassionate energy that is expended by nurses outweighs the restorative processes and in which the ability to recover has been lost; it is the negative aspect of helping that can be related to the actual provision of care, the environment, colleagues, or beliefs about self.[76,77] Burnout, on the other hand, relates to work-related hopelessness. *Burnout* is the inability to cope with job stress, which produces feelings of inefficacy.[78] *Moral distress* arises when one must act in a way that contradicts personal values and beliefs; *moral fatigue* is the consequence of continued moral distress.[79,80] For example, nurses might act in a way that is contrary to personal and professional values or be able to translate moral choices into action. This creates anguish; the consequences can be profound and have lasting effects.[79] Nurses who appear to be at a higher risk for compassion fatigue include those who are younger, have a history of personal trauma, and have not worked through issues related to trauma; those who have large caseloads or long hours; and those who are already experiencing professional burnout, have inadequate training in effective communication, and lack adequate collegiate and personal support systems.[75]

### Coping Strategies

Coping strategies, including self-care, are key to prevention of compassion fatigue. Integrating self-care activities, including self-compassion and mindfulness-based strategies, into professional workloads is not typically part of professional training, nor is it explicitly part of one's job description. If nurses do not care for themselves, they will be unable to sustain care for others [81,82]

### Moral Distress

Moral distress is often created in situations in which nurses participate in activities that are perceived as medically futile. Providing futile care undermines the core of the professional practice of nursing. One of the most crucial elements in dealing with moral distress is knowing *what* support is available and *how* to navigate the system in place. Ethics committees are one source of support and serve to assist in resolving complicated ethical problems that affect the care and treatment of patients within healthcare organizations. The Joint Commission on Accreditation of Healthcare Organizations requires hospitals and other healthcare organizations to have a mechanism in place to address ethical issues in the provision of patient care. Healthcare organizations have different mechanisms by which to address ethical issues. It is the responsibility of all nurses to know what resources are available in their organization and how to access them. Just as preventive ethics should be used before an ethical dilemma arises, so should they be used to guide nursing practice before a crisis occurs.

## Summary

There will always be ethical dilemmas in palliative care and end-of-life care. The answers to the dilemma will not always be obvious or easily identified. It is often in states of uncertainty that serious wrongs occur. As we partner in the care of patient and their families with advanced illness, difficult decision may have to be made. Nurses play a crucial role in facilitating these discussion. A grounding in ethical principles, excellent communication skills, and self-reflection will enable them to fulfill this crucial role.

## References

1. Bishop, AH, Scudder, JR. *The Practical, Moral, and Personal Sense of Nursing: A Phenomenological Philosophy of Practice.* Albany, NY: State University of New York Press; 1990.

2. Honderich T. *The Oxford Guide to Philosophy.* 2nd ed. Oxford, UK: Oxford University Press; 2005.

3. Gert B. *Morality: Its Nature and Justification.* Oxford, UK: Oxford University Press; 2005.
4. Koehn D. *Rethinking Feminist Ethics.* New York: Routledge; 2001.
5. Nodding N. *Caring.* Berkeley, CA: University of California Press; 1984.
6. Mullan F, Ficklen E, Rubin K, Eds. *Narrative Matters.* Baltimore: Johns Hopkins University Press, 2006.
7. Fry S. The role of caring in a theory of nursing ethics. In: Holmes HB, Purdy LM, eds. *Feminist Perspectives in Medical Ethics.* Indianapolis, IN: Indiana University Press; 1992:93–106.
8. Sudore RL, Fried TR. Redefining the "planning" in advance care planning: preparing for end-of-life decision making. *Ann Intern Med.* 2010;153(4):256–261.
9. Foglia MB, Fox E, Chanko B, Bottrell MM. Preventive ethics: addressing ethics quality gaps on a systems level. *Joint Commission Journal on Quality and Patient Safety.* 2012;38(3):103–111.
10. Mack JW, Weeks JC, Wright AA, Block SD, Prigerson HG. End-of-life discussions, goal attainment, and distress at the end of life: predictors and outcomes of receipt of care consistent with preferences. *J Clin Oncol.* 2010;28(7):120311208.
11. Mack JW, Cronin A, Keating NL, et al. Associations between end-of-life discussion characteristics and care received near death: a prospective cohort study. *J Clin Oncol.* 2012;30(35):4387–4395.
12. Detering KM, Hancock AD, Reade MC, Silvester W. The impact of advance care planning on end of life care in elderly patients: randomised controlled trial. *BMJ.* 2010;340:c1345.
13. Billings JA. The need for safeguards in advance care planning. *J Gen Intern Med.* 2012;27(5):595–600.
14. Yung VY, Walling AM, Min L, Wenger NS, Ganz DA. Documentation of advance care planning for community-dwelling elders. *J Palliat Med.* 2010;13(7):861–867.
15. Aging With Dignity. *Five Wishes.* http://www.agingwithdignity.org/five-wishes-states.php. Accessed August 17, 2015.
16. Hickman SE, Nelson CA, Perrin NA, et al. A comparison of methods to communicate treatment preferences in nursing facilities: traditional practices versus the physician orders for life-sustaining treatment program. *J Am Geriatr Soc.* 2010;58(7):1241–1248.
17. Citko J, Moss AH, Carley M, Tolle S. *The National POLST Paradigm Initiative.* 2nd ed., #178. *J Palliat Med.* 2011;14(2):241–242.
18. Araw AC, Araw AM, Pekmezaris R, et al. Medical orders for life-sustaining treatment: is it time yet? *Palliat Support Care.* 2014;12(2):101–105.
19. Bomba PA, Kemp M, Black JS. POLST: an improvement over traditional advance directives. *Cleve Clin J Med.* 2012;79(7):457–464.
20. Center to Advance Palliative Care. *Fast Facts.* https://www.capc.org/fast-facts/. Accessed August 17, 2015.
21. National Consensus Project. http://www.nationalconsensusproject.org/Guidelines_Download2.aspx. Accessed August 17, 2015.
22. Ehlenbach WJ, Barnato AE, Curtis JR, et al. Epidemiologic study of in-hospital cardiopulmonary resuscitation in the elderly. *N Engl J Med.* 2009;361(1):22–31.
23. Jones GK, Brewer KL, Garrison HG. Public expectations of survival following cardiopulmonary resuscitation. *Acad Emerg Med.* 2000;7(1):48–53.

24. ECC Committee. Subcommittees and Task Forces of the American Heart Association. 2005 American Heart Association guidelines for cardiopulmonary resuscitation and emergency cardiovascular care. *Circulation*. 2005;112(24 Suppl):1–203.

25. American College of Emergency Physicians. "Do Not Attempt Resuscitation" Orders in the Out of Hospital Setting. http://www.acep.org/Clinical---Practice-Management/-Do-Not-Attempt-Resuscitation--Orders-in-the-Out-of-Hospital-Setting/. Accessed August 17, 2015.

26. Kirchhoff K, Spuhler V, Walker L, et al. Intensive care nurses' experiences with end-of-life care. *Am J Crit Care*. 2000;9(1):36–42.

27. Post LF, Blustein J, Dubler NN. *Handbook for Health Care Ethics Committees*. Baltimore, MD: Johns Hopkins University Press; 2007.

28. Zettel-Watson L, Ditto PH, Danks JH, Smucker WD. Actual and perceived gender differences in the accuracy of surrogate decisions about life-sustaining medical treatment among older spouses. *Death Stud*. 2008;32(3):273–290.

29. Shalowitz DI, Garrett-Mayer E, Wendler D. The accuracy of surrogate decision makers: a systematic review. *Arch Intern Med*. 2006;166(5):493.

30. Beauchamp TL, Childress JF. *Principles of Biomedical Ethics*. 6th ed. New York, NY: Oxford University Press; 2008.

31. New Jersey Superior Court, Morris County, NJ. In the matter of Karen Quinlan: the complete legal briefs, court proceedings, and decision in the Superior Court of New Jersey. *Univ Publ Am*. 1975;1.

32. Nancy Beth Cruzan, by her parents and co-guardians, Lester L. Cruzan et ux. v. Director, Missouri Department of Health et al. 497, US 261, 1990.

33. Greer GW, Judge C. In re: the guardianship of Theresa Marie Schiavo, incapacitated. Michael Schiavo, petitioner, vs. Robert Schindler and Mary Schindler, respondents. File No.90-2908-GD-003. Fla. 6th Judicial Circuit, February 25, 2005.

34. Sampson EL, Candy B, Jones L. Enteral tube feeding for older people with advanced dementia. *Cochrane Database Syst Rev*. 2009;(2):CD007209.

35. Geppert CM, Andrews MR, Druyan ME. Ethical issues in artificial nutrition and hydration: a review. *JPEN J Parenter Enteral Nutr*. 2010;34(1):79–88.

36. Zerwekh JV. The dehydration question. *Nursing 2012*. 1983;13(1):47–56.

37. Teno JM, Gozalo P, Mitchell SL, et al. Feeding tubes and the prevention or healing of pressure ulcers. *Arch Intern Med*. 2012;172(9):697–701.

38. Palecek EJ, Teno JM, Casarett DJ, et al. Comfort feeding only: a proposal to bring clarity to decision-making regarding difficulty with eating for persons with advanced dementia. *J Am Geriatr Soc*. 2010;58(3):580–584.

39. Teno JM, Mitchell SL, Gozalo PL, et al. Hospital characteristics associated with feeding tube placement in nursing home residents with advanced cognitive impairment. *JAMA*. 2010;303(6):544–550.

40. Moynihan T, Kelly DG, Fisch MJ. To feed or not to feed: Is that the right question? *J Clin Oncol*. 2005;23(25):6256–6259.

41. Morita T, Shima Y, Miyashita M, Kimura R, Adachi I. Physician- and nurse-reported effects of intravenous hydration therapy on symptoms of terminally ill patients with cancer. *J Palliat Med*. 2004;7(5):683–693.

42. Hanson LC, Garrett JM, Lewis C, et al. Physicians' expectations of benefit from tube feeding. *J Palliat Med*. 2008;11(8):1130–1134.

43. Washington State Legislature. The Washington Death With Dignity Act. http://apps.leg.wa.gov/RCW/default.aspx?cite=70.245. Updated 2008. Accessed August 17, 2015.

44. Emanuel EJ, Fairclough DL, Emanuel LL. Attitudes and desires related to euthanasia and physician-assisted suicide among terminally ill patients and their caregivers. *JAMA:.* 2000;284(19):2460–2468.

45. O'Mahony S, Goulet J, Kornblith A, et al. Desire for hastened death, cancer pain and depression: teport of a longitudinal observational study. *J Pain Symptom Manage.* 2005;29(5):446–457.

46. van Bruchem-van de Scheur GG, van der Arend AJ, Huijer Abu-Saad H, et al. Euthanasia and assisted suicide in Dutch hospitals: the role of nurses. *J Clin Nurs.* 2008;17(12):1618–1626.

47. Ganzini L, Goy ER, Dobscha SK. Prevalence of depression and anxiety in patients requesting physicians' aid in dying: Cross sectional survey. *BMJ.* 2008;337:a1682.

48. Quill T, Arnold RM. Evaluating requests for hastened death # 156. *J Palliat Med.* 2008;11(8):1151-1152.

49. Hudson PL, Schofield P, Kelly B, et al. Responding to desire to die statements from patients with advanced disease: recommendations for health professionals. *Palliat Med.* 2006;20(7):703–710.

50. Mond HG, Irwin M, Ector H, Proclemer A. The world survey of cardiac pacing and cardioverter-defibrillators: calendar year 2005 an international cardiac pacing and electrophysiology society (ICPES) project. *Pacing Clin Electrophysiol.* 2008;31(9):1202–1212.

51. Mueller PS, Jenkins SM, Bramstedt KA, Hayes DL. Deactivating implanted cardiac devices in terminally ill patients: practices and attitudes. *Pacing Clin Electrophysiol* 2008;31(5):560–568.

52. Hansson SO. Implant ethics. *J Med Ethics.* 2005;31(9):519–525.

53. Kramer DB, Kesselheim AS, Brock DW, Maisel WH. Ethical and legal views of physicians regarding deactivation of cardiac implantable electrical devices: a quantitative assessment. *Heart Rhythm.* 2010;7(11):1537–1542.

54. Grady KL, Shinn JA. Care of patients with circulatory assist devices. In: Moser DK, Riegel B, ed. *Cardiac Nursing.* Philadelphia: Mosby; 2008:977–987.

55. Rizzieri AG, Verheijde JL, Rady MY, McGregor JL. Ethical challenges with the left ventricular assist device as a destination therapy. *Philos Ethics Humanit Med.* 2008;3:20.

56. Swetz KM, Ottenberg AL, Freeman MR, Mueller PS. Palliative care and end-of-life issues in patients treated with left ventricular assist devices as destination therapy. *Curr Heart Fail Rep.* 2011;8(3):212–218.

57. Swetz KM, Freeman MR, AbouEzzeddine OF, et al. Palliative medicine consultation for preparedness planning in patients receiving left ventricular assist devices as destination therapy. *Mayo Clin Proc.* 2011;86(6):493–500.

58. Chapman E, Parameshwar J, Jenkins D, Large S, Tsui S. Psychosocial issues for patients with ventricular assist devices: a qualitative pilot study. *Am J Crit Care.* 2007;16(1):72–81.

59. Zambroski CH, Combs P, Cronin SN, Pfeffer C. Edgar Allan Poe, "The Pit and the Pendulum," and ventricular assist devices. *Crit Care Nurse.* 2009;29(6):29–39.

60. Lampert R, Hayes DL, Annas GJ, et al. HRS expert consensus statement on the management of cardiovascular implantable electronic devices

(CIEDs) in patients nearing end of life or requesting removal. *Heart Rhythm.* 2010;7(7):1008–1026.

61. Quill TE, Lo B, Brock DW, Meisel A. Last-resort options for palliative sedation. *Ann Intern Med.* 2009;151(6):421–424.

62. Maltoni M, Scarpi E, Rosati M, et al. Palliative sedation in end-of-life care and survival: a systematic review. *J Clin Oncol.* 2012;30(12):1378–1383.

63. Cassell EJ, Rich BA. Intractable end-of-life suffering and the ethics of palliative sedation. *Pain Med.* 2010;11(3):435–438.

64. Claessens P, Menten J, Schotsmans P, Broeckaert B. Palliative sedation: a review of the research literature. *J Pain Symptom Manage.* 2008;36(3):310–333.

65. Bernat JL. Medical futility. *Neurocrit Care.* 2005;2(2):198–205.

66. Caplan AL. Little hope for medical futility. *Mayo Clin Proc.* 2012;87(11):1040–1041.

67. Moseley KL, Silveira MJ, Goold SD. Futility in evolution. *Clin Geriatr Med.* 2005;21(1):211–222.

68. Wicclair MR. Medical futility: A conceptual and ethical analysis. In DeGrazia D, Mappes TA, Brand-Ballard J, eds. Biomedical Ethics. Vol. 6, 7th ed. New York, NY: McGraw-Hill; 2006:345–349.

69. von Gruenigen VE, Daly BJ. Futility: clinical decisions at the end-of-life in women with ovarian cancer. *Gynecol Oncol.* 2005;97(2):638–644.

70. Daly BJ. An indecent proposal: withholding cardiopulmonary resuscitation. *Am J Crit Care.* 2008;17(4):377–380.

71. Wilkinson DJ, Savulescu J. Knowing when to stop: futility in the intensive care unit. *Curr Opin Anaesthesiol* 2011;24(2):160.

72. White DB, Pope TM. The courts, futility, and the ends of medicine. *JAMA.* 2012;307(2):151–152.

73. Ferrell BR, Coyle N. *The Nature of Suffering and the Goals of Nursing.* Oxford, UK: Oxford University Press; 2008.

74. Ferrell BR. Understanding the moral distress of nurses witnessing medically futile care. *Oncol Nurs Forum.* 2006;33(5):922–930.

75. Aycock N, Boyle D. Interventions to manage compassion fatigue in oncology nursing. *Clin J Oncol Nurs.* 2009;13(2):183–191.

76. Coetzee SK, Klopper HC. Compassion fatigue within nursing practice: a concept analysis. *Nurs Health Sci.* 2010;12(2):235–243.

77. Figley CR. *Treating Compassion Fatigue.* New York, NY: Routledge, Psychology Press; 2002.

78. Alkema K, Linton JM, Davies R. A study of the relationship between self-care, compassion satisfaction, compassion fatigue, and burnout among hospice professionals. *J Soc Work End Life Palliat Care.* 2008;4(2):101-119.

79. Wiegand DL, Funk M. Consequences of clinical situations that cause critical care nurses to experience moral distress. *Nurs Ethics.* 2012;19(4):479–487

80. Varcoe C, Pauly B, Storch J, et al. Nurses' perceptions of and responses to morally distressing situations. *Nurs Ethics.* 2012;19(4):488–500.

81. Clark E. Self-care as best practice in palliative care. In: Altilio T, Otis-Green S, eds. Oxford Textbook of Palliative Social Work. New York, NY: Oxford University Press; 2011:771–777.

82. Cacciatore J, Flint M. ATTEND: toward a mindfulness-based bereavement care model. *Death Stud.* 2012;36:61–82.

# Chapter 2

# Palliative Care and Requests for Assistance in Dying

Deborah L. Volker

> ### Key Points
> - Palliative care nurses encounter patient and family questions, concerns, and requests for assisted dying.
> - Withholding and withdrawing life-sustaining measures, administering palliative sedation, and providing pain relief are not acts of assisted dying.
> - Individuals with life-limiting disease who may consider assisted dying include those experiencing unrelieved pain, depression, hopelessness, psychological distress, spiritual distress, poor social support, poor quality of life, or perception of being a burden on others.
> - Nurses should respond to requests for assisted dying in a manner that reflects professional guidelines and a sense of advocacy for patient rights for quality end-of-life care.

## Overview of Palliative Care and Requests for Assistance in Dying

The concept of palliative care, as described by the World Health Organization, is in direct conflict with the idea of deliberately hastening a person's death through the practice of assisted dying. Indeed, palliative care "intends neither to hasten nor postpone death."[1] Yet patients may be fearful of the extreme discomfort they anticipate as death approaches, or they may simply want some certainty as to the timing or circumstances of death. Nurses who care for patients with life-limiting disease encounter patient and family questions, concerns, and requests for assisted dying. Receiving such a request can represent a morally troubling dilemma in which there is uncertainty about how best to respond. The purpose of this chapter is to review the ethical and legal status of assisted dying, summarize empirical findings regarding both professional and lay opinions and experiences with assisted dying, and offer guidelines for responding to requests for assisted dying.

## What Is Assisted Dying?

- The term *assisted dying* is typically used to describe an action in which an individual's death is intentionally hastened by the administration of a drug or other lethal substance. This may take the form of either assisted suicide or euthanasia.

- *Assisted suicide* indicates that "the means to end a patient's life is provided to the patient (i.e. a lethal dose of medication) with knowledge of the patient's intention. Unlike euthanasia, in assisted suicide, someone makes the means of death available, but does not act as the direct agent of death."[2] Of note, in states where assisted suicide is legal, prescriptions for lethal doses of medication, not weapons, are provided to qualified patients.

- *Euthanasia,* "often called 'mercy killing', is the act of putting to death someone suffering from a painful and prolonged illness or injury. Euthanasia means that someone other than the patient commits an action with the intent to end the patient's life, for example injecting a patient with a lethal dose of medication."[2] Such an action can be voluntary (e.g., requested by a competent individual) or involuntary (administered without the individual's knowledge or consent).

Distinguishing between "assisted dying" and actions allowing a patient to die comfortably:

- Intent and causation are the key concepts that differentiate the two actions.

## What Is Withholding or Withdrawing Life-Sustaining Measures?

Withholding and withdrawing life-sustaining measures are actions designed to not interfere with the natural trajectory of an illness. That is, life-sustaining measures such as artificial ventilation, renal dialysis, cardiopulmonary resuscitation, or artificial nutrition and hydration are withheld or stopped; the patient subsequently dies because of the effects of disease. In this instance, the intent of the action is to allow a natural death, and the cause of death is the underlying illness. In contrast, in assisted dying, the intent of the action is to hasten death, and the cause of death is the lethal drug or other means administered to end life.

The public and some healthcare providers continue to be confused about the definition and intent of palliative care versus actions designed to deliberately hasten death. For example, in a lay magazine article,[3] palliative care was characterized as the "new stealth euthanasia" that is changing medical care in the United States "from lifesaving medicine to life rationing [sic] medicine (p. 3)." Palliative care physicians, nurses, and other practitioners may experience this sentiment in the clinical setting.[4]

Goldstein and colleagues conducted a survey of the frequency of formal accusations of murder and euthanasia against 663 hospice and palliative care physicians.[4] Findings revealed that more than half of the sample had patient family members or other healthcare providers misinterpret the study participants' palliative care practices as murder or euthanasia. The most commonly reported misperceived actions included the use of opiates for symptom control and the use of palliative and sedating medications during discontinuation of mechanical ventilation to prevent suffering. Clearly, efforts to educate the public and healthcare providers about the moral and legal status of palliative care practices must be intensified. Knowledge of the principle of double effect can be useful here.

### The Principle of Double Effect

Some practitioners worry that administration of sufficient doses of pain medication and other drugs designed to relieve suffering may hasten death and therefore may constitute assisted dying.

This is *not* an action of assisted dying. It does not qualify as assisted dying because the intent is to relieve suffering, even though there may be a foreseen possibility that the medications could result in a hastened death. This is an example of the ethical principle of double effect in which a good effect (relief of pain or other symptoms) is the goal despite the possibility of an unintended, harmful effect (a hastened death). The principle of double effect includes the following features:

- The act is morally good or neutral.
- Good effect is intended.
- Bad effect is foreseen as a potential.
- Bad effect is not the means to the good effect.
- Proportionality—the good that one is trying to achieve must outweigh the bad that could happen. This ratio may change based on goals of care.

## Ethical and Legal Issues

The ethical and legal issues associated with assisted dying have been well described. Those who believe that assisted dying is ethical cite the following points[5-7]:

- It allows patients the right to determine their own fate (autonomy).
- It enables the relief of untenable suffering.
- It allows patients to maintain control over the end of their life.
- It ensure equity: patients not dependent on life support do not have the same access to ending life as someone who can deliberately end life by discontinuing a respirator.

Those who believe assisted dying is unethical worry that the practice will do the following:

- Erode trust in healthcare professions
- Deny the sanctity of human life
- Discourage efforts to make palliative care available to all
- Initiate a "slippery slope" toward euthanasia
- Pressure the vulnerable, underserved, disabled, or disenfranchised to take a quick way out with death

Historically, the healthcare professions' ethical codes and position statements uniformly opposed legal assisted dying. However, more recent trends reveal that a few organizations are neutral on the topic, take no formal stand but advise members as to their ethical responsibilities as patient advocates, or support patients who choose legal assisted dying.[8-10]

Nursing organizations continue to oppose assisted dying. Table 2.1 summarizes their relevant position statements.

- Euthanasia is illegal throughout the United States, although physician-assisted death is legal in five states.
- The Netherlands, Belgium, and Luxembourg allow both euthanasia and assisted suicide under certain circumstances.[11]
- Switzerland is unique in that it (1) allows assisted suicide to be facilitated by nonphysicians (although a physician must prescribe the lethal medication, nonphysician volunteers may provide assistance, such as connecting patients with physicians who are willing to prescribe a lethal drug, providing an apartment for the suicide, and so forth); (2) allows foreign citizens to engage in the practice within its borders; and (3) does not require that a person have a particular illness or prognosis.[12]

Worldwide, the Netherlands has had more experience with the practice of euthanasia than any other country. Euthanasia was legally sanctioned through a series of court decisions in the Netherlands beginning in the 1970s; euthanasia and physician-assisted suicide were legalized in 2002 by the Dutch parliament.[13] Controversy exists as to whether increasing tolerance of these practices by physicians and the public has led to an increase in their use and less emphasis on palliative and hospice care.[14] Onwuteaka-Philipsen and colleagues studied trends in end-of-life practices in the Netherlands from 1990 to 2010 through a repeated cross-sectional survey.[11] Although the overall incidence of deaths due to physician-assisted suicide had not changed between 1990 and 2010, the incidence of euthanasia did increase between 2005 and 2010. Over the study period, far fewer deaths were due to physician-assisted death than euthanasia (e.g., 21 versus 475 in 2010). Other trends included the following:

- An increase in the use of deep sedation before death
- An increase in the use of intensified strategies to address pain and other symptoms at the end of life
- A decrease in the frequency of ending life without a patient's request.

The researchers speculated that these trends may reflect an increased interest in palliative care and that regulations enacted in 2002 may have facilitated more open discussions between patients and physicians about end-of-life care. However, the study did not evaluate quality of end-of-life care and hospice use, nor did it obtain views of patients or family members.

Assisted suicide was legalized in Oregon in 1997 with the passage of the Death with Dignity Act by two citizen referenda separated by 3 years. This Act allows a terminally ill person to obtain a prescription for a lethal dose of medication with the prescribing physician's understanding that the intent of the medication is to end life.

Table 2.1 Position Statements of Nursing Organizations Relevant to Patient Requests for Assisted Dying

| Organization | Title | Key Points |
|---|---|---|
| American Nurses Association (ANA)[2] | Euthanasia, Assisted Suicide, and Aid in Dying | The ANA "prohibits nurses' participation in assisted suicide and euthanasia because these acts are in direct violation of Code of Ethics for Nurses With Interpretive Statements (p. 1). Nurses are obliged to provide compassionate, competent care that respects patients rights while also upholding nursing practice standards focused on "chronic, debilitating illness and the end of life" (p. 1). Although the ANA recognizes that some nurses practice in locales where assisted suicide is legal, the ANA Center for Ethics and Human Rights offers support and consultation services to them regarding their professional responsibilities. |
| American Nurses Association[18] | Registered Nurses' Roles and Responsibilities in Providing Expert Care and Counseling at the End of Life | "Nurses, individually and collectively, have an obligation to provide comprehensive and compassionate end-of-life care, including the promotion of comfort, relief of pain, and support for patients, families, and their surrogates when a decision has been made to forgo life-sustaining treatments" (p. 2). "While nurses should make every effort to provide aggressive pain control and symptom relief for patients at the end of life, it is never ethically permissible for a nurse to act by omission or commission, including, but not limited to medication administration, with the intention of ending a patient's life" (p. 2). |
| American Society for Pain Management Nurses[19] | ASPMN Position Statement on Assisted Suicide | Supports the ANA position against nurses' participation in assisted suicide or euthanasia and "supports improved access for pain management services and other modalities that will benefit terminally ill patients and their families" (p. 1) |
| Hospice and Palliative Nurses Association[20] | Legalization of Assisted Suicide | "Opposes the legalization of assisted suicide" and "affirms the value of aggressive and comprehensive end-of-life care" (p. 2). "Advises nurses practicing in states where assisted suicide is legal that they have the moral and legal right to refuse to be involved in the care of patients requesting assisted suicide" but must remain nonjudgmental and transfer the patient's care to other nurses (p. 2) |

(continued)

### Table 2.1 (Continued)

| Organization | Title | Key Points |
|---|---|---|
| Hospice and Palliative Nurses Association[21] | *Role of the Nurse When Hastened Death Is Requested* | "Both patient's rights and nurses' values should be respected" (p. 2). Nurses should assess patient requests for hastened death, provide aggressive palliative care, and "share information about health choices that are legal and support the patient and family regardless of the decision that is made" (p. 2). |
| Oncology Nursing Society[22] | *Nurses' Responsibility to Patients Requesting Assistance in Hastening Death* | Does not support actions intended to hasten death but "supports continued efforts to improve compassionate, evidence-based care for the dying and encourages continued dialogue on any and all ethical dilemmas." Responses to requests for hastened death should "prompt a frank discussion of the rationale for the request, a thorough and nonjudgmental multidisciplinary assessment of the patient's unmet needs, and prompt and intensive intervention for previously unrecognized or unmet needs" (p. 1). |
| Oregon Nurses Association[23] | *ONA Provides Guidance on Nurses' Dilemma* | Does not support or oppose legalized assisted suicide. "If the patient inquires about the option of assisted suicide, one of the roles of the nurse, as health care provider, is to share relevant information about health choices that are legal and to support the patient and family regardless of the decision the patient makes." Provides guidelines for acceptable practices for nurses who choose to be, or not to be, involved with a patient who requests legal assistance to hasten death. |
| Vermont State Nurses' Association (VSNA)[24] | *VSNA Position Statement on Physician-Assisted Suicide* | "Opposes the legalization of physician assisted suicide and believes that the nurse should not participate in assisted suicide" (p. 12). Identifies key components of "dignified and humane end-of life care" and believes that "the focus on physician assisted suicide distracts attention and resources from the real work of helping our patients live meaningful lives in their final days" (p. 12). |

Eligible patients must meet several criteria; they must be at least 18 years of age, an Oregon resident, capable of making healthcare decisions, and diagnosed with a terminal illness that will cause death within 6 months. The patient who requests a prescription must make two oral requests (separated by at least 15 days) to his or her physician and provide a written request that is signed in the presence of two witnesses. The prescribing physician and a consulting physician must confirm the diagnosis and prognosis and determine whether the patient is capable of making the decision. If either physician believes the patient's judgment is in question, the patient must be referred for a psychological examination. The prescribing physician must also discuss alternatives to assisted suicide (comfort care, hospice care, and pain control) with the patient and must request (but not require) that the patient notify next of kin of his or her plans.[12,15]

The Act was challenged in 2001 by the U.S. Attorney General, who asserted that physicians who prescribe lethal doses of drugs are violating federal laws regarding controlled substances. The U.S. Supreme Court ruled in 2006 that the Attorney General does not have the authority to determine what constitutes a legitimate medical practice and that individual states retain this responsibility.[16] Hence, the Oregon Act remains in place, and physicians may continue to prescribe controlled substances for the purpose of hastening death. Only about 1 in every 1000 Oregonians who die uses assisted suicide as an end-of-life option.[17]

Since Oregon legalized assisted suicide, four additional states have approved the practice. In 2008, voters in Washington State approved a Death With Dignity Act that is modeled after the Oregon law. Although Montana does not have a similar statute, the Montana Supreme Court ruled that physician-assisted suicide was not illegal in 2009,[5] which paved the way for legal patient access to the practice. In 2013, Vermont's state legislature and governor approved a law that allows physician-assisted suicide. Although the law has safeguards similar to those in Oregon and Washington, after a 3-year period of governmental restrictions expires in 2016, prescribing practices of physicians who write legal prescriptions for assisted suicide will become more private and guided by professional practice standards that guide physician conduct.[25] Most recently, in October 2015. the Governor of California signed into law the "End of Life Act" protecting patients' right to choose doctor-assisted death.

## Who Wants Access to Assisted Dying and Why?

It is not unusual for terminally ill people to desire a hastened death. People who have life-limiting diseases such as cancer, degenerative neurologic disorders, or end-stage cardiovascular or renal disease have been identified as individuals who may be interested in access to assisted dying. Various studies have revealed characteristics of those who have expressed a desire for hastened death. Ferrand and colleagues conducted a national survey of palliative care departments in France to describe the evolution of requests for hastened death among their patients.[26] Of the 342 teams who responded, 783 descriptions of requests were provided.

Characteristics of patients who desired to hasten their death included the following:

- Had a cancer diagnosis (72%)
- Were terminally ill (68%)
- Had controlled pain (52%)
- Had a feeding impairment (65%)
- Were incontinent (49%)
- Had a motor impairment (54%)

Less than 4% had uncontrolled pain, which may have been a reflection of care management by palliative specialists. The most commonly reported patient perceptions of their concerns included "a fear of presenting an unbearable image of oneself" (50%) and a fear of becoming a burden on family (46%).

Cancer is a major risk factor for an affected person's interest in suicide. In a case-control study of suicide risk in older Americans with medical illnesses, cancer was the only illness that was associated with a higher risk for suicide.[27] The study authors conjectured that contributing factors may have included advanced disease and its treatment or social responses to progressive disease such as intractable pain, poor prognosis, use of higher doses of analgesics, or social isolation. The study focused on analysis of actual suicides and did not capture desire for suicide that was not enacted.

Historically, risk for suicide in cancer patients has been associated with end-stage disease, depression, or hopelessness.[28] Further, in a study of the clinical features of suicidality in patients with advanced cancer, patients who were more likely to have suicidal thoughts (9% of the sample) than those who did not were non-Hispanic whites, reported no religious affiliation, and were diagnosed with a current panic disorder or post-traumatic stress disorder.[29] However, Walker and colleagues surveyed approximately 3,000 outpatients with cancer to determine prevalence of suicidal thoughts.[30] About 8% reported suicidal thoughts. Emotional distress, substantial pain, and older age were associated with suicidal ideation in this group of patients. This finding suggests that assessment for suicidal risk in cancer patients must go beyond those with terminal illness.

Patients with amyotrophic lateral sclerosis (ALS) are at higher risk than the general population for interest in hastening death through physician-assisted suicide or euthanasia. Typically, contributing variables include severe, advanced-stage disease, treatment ineffectiveness, and increasing dependence on caregivers.[31] However, in a 40-year, case-controlled study of suicide in Sweden, people with ALS had a sixfold increased risk for suicide than the general population, but the risk was higher in earlier stages of the disease.[31] The study investigators hypothesized that severe emotional burden associated with a new diagnosis of ALS and physical inability to perform suicide at later stages of disease could have accounted for their findings. In the Netherlands, death due to euthanasia is more common among people with ALS than with a cancer diagnosis.[32]

Experience with legal assisted dying in Oregon reveals another picture. During the first 15 years of the Death With Dignity Act, 673 patients took lethal medications to end their lives, whereas 1,050 Oregonians received prescriptions for assisted dying under the Act.[33]

Characteristics of Oregonians who died from assisted dying include the following:
- Older age (median: 71 years)
- White race and college-level education
- Diagnosis of either cancer or ALS
- Enrollment in hospice care
- Private or governmental health insurance

The most common end-of-life concerns voiced included the following:
- Loss of autonomy
- Decreased ability to participate in enjoyable activities
- Loss of dignity[33]

## Perspectives of Families and Healthcare Providers

Various studies of Oregon patients, families, and healthcare providers' attitudes and experiences with assisted suicide have unfolded since the enactment of the Death With Dignity Act. In a study of the quality of death and dying in patients who requested physician-assisted death, Smith and colleagues examined the perspectives of family members of patients who had received prescriptions for assisted dying, patients who sought but did not receive such prescriptions, and patients who did not request assisted dying.[34]

When comparing symptom control, connectedness with others, existential issues, preparedness for death, and global indicators of quality of life and death, the researchers[34] concluded that "the quality of death experienced by those who received lethal prescriptions is no worse than those not pursuing physician assisted death, and in some areas is rated by family members as better" (p. 445). These areas included symptom control and preparedness for death.

## Reasons for a Request for Aid in Dying

Given that data reported to the Oregon Public Health Division regarding patients' experiences with the Death With Dignity Act are provided by physicians, Ganzini and colleagues took a different approach and investigated Oregonians' reasons for requesting physician aid in dying.[35] In a survey of 56 individuals who had expressed interest in physician-assisted dying, the most important reasons for their interest included the following:
- Concerns about loss of control over independence
- Circumstances of death
- Ability to care for self
- Concern about physical discomfort in the future

The authors concluded that study results should prompt healthcare providers to address patient requests for assisted dying by addressing autonomy issues and worries about symptom control as the end of life unfolds.

Despite access to legal assisted dying, or perhaps because of it, Oregon is a national leader in improving planning for and delivery of quality of end-of-life care. Oregon is among only 8 states to receive an "A" grade for access to palliative care[36] and among 13 states to receive an "A" grade for the quality of its policies that affect pain treatment.[37] The Oregon Physicians Orders for Life Sustaining Treatment (POLST) program was created 20 years ago to implement a system that captures a patient's treatment preferences and electronically records them as medical records accessible across care settings.[38] The population of focus is those with advanced or chronic progressive illness or frailty. Now codified by Oregon state law, POLST has served as a model program nationally and has been adopted by 15 states, with laws in 28 other states under development.[38]

## What Do Studies Reveal About Nurses and Assisted Dying?

Given their pivotal role in providing palliative care, nurses may encounter patient requests for assisted dying. Both survey and interview studies have captured nurses' experiences with receiving requests for assisted dying. For example, in a classic study conducted by Matzo and Emanuel,[39] the investigators surveyed 441 New England oncology nurses and discovered that 30% had received requests for assisted suicide, 1% had engaged in assisted suicide, and 4.5% had injected a drug to intentionally end a patient's life. In a national survey of more than 2,333 nurses,[40] 23% had received patient requests for assistance with obtaining a lethal prescription, and 22% had patients who requested that they be injected with a lethal dose of medication.

Harvath and colleagues[41] interviewed 20 nurses and social workers regarding their experiences with patients who wished to hasten death and found their experience presented opportunities to discuss patient concerns and fears about the dying process and to improve symptom management strategies. These experiences, however, also presented nurses and social worker with a conflict between respecting patients' autonomy and honoring their own commitment to uphold the goals of hospice care.

In a subsequent study of policies developed by 56 Oregon hospices to manage patient requests for legal assisted dying under the Death With Dignity Act, researchers found that these policies reflected ambivalence between a commitment to care for all patients regardless of interest in assisted dying and the traditional goals of hospice care to neither hasten death nor prolong life.[42]

The question of what constitutes participation (or not) in assisted dying manifested in a variety of ways, as follows:
- Policies ranged from providing information about the law to patients exploring patient requests for hastened death to encouraging patient contact with their physicians.
- Many of the policies reflected an emphasis on the importance of maintaining neutrality during patient discussion.
- Almost all of the policies contained a prohibition against assistance with a lethal medication: "Hospice X will not provide, pay for, deliver, administer or assist with medications intended for physician-assisted dying (p. 233)," nor did hospitals allow their staff to assist the patient to self-administer the medication.[42]

Nonetheless, during the investigators' site visits at participating hospices, some nurses revealed that they would "attend" a patient during an assisted death but not while "on duty." Washington nurses are now investigating issues associated with implementation of legal assisted dying.

Two years after implementation of the Washington State Death With Dignity Act, Jablonski[43] and Clymin[44] and their colleagues surveyed 582 members of the Washington State Nurses Association to determine their knowledge about the new law. Most of the respondents accurately understood some components of the law, including eligibility for assisted dying, physicians' and institutions' rights to refuse to participate, and restrictions limiting prescribing practices for lethal doses of medications to physicians only. Conversely, less than half of the respondents could accurately answer 9 of 25 knowledge items, ranging from inaccurately specifying a requirement for an interdisciplinary team evaluation of assisted dying request to misunderstanding employing institution or facility rights regarding the restriction of assisted dying practices. Only 7% of the respondents had received education about the new law when it was first enacted, and many expressed concern about their lack of knowledge regarding the Act.

In a survey of 532 Dutch inpatient nurses, investigators examined the role of nurses in managing patient requests for euthanasia or assisted suicide, the decision-making process, and the administration of lethal drugs.[45] Findings revealed the following:

- Patients often speak with their nurses first about their wishes for hastened death.
- Nurses respond by explaining legal requirements, hospital policies, and opportunities for palliative care.
- Most nurses reported discussing patient requests with physician colleagues.
- Notably, nurses administered a lethal drug with or without a physician present to 22 patients. Dutch law limits the administration of euthanatics to physicians only.

# How Should Nurses Respond to Requests for Assisted Dying?

Of the myriad communication skills expected of nurses, responding to requests for assisted dying can be the most difficult. Not surprisingly, many nurses feel ill equipped to address a patient's interest in suicide. According to Valente,[46] barriers to appropriate nursing management of suicide risk include communication issues, such as not knowing how to respond; personal judgments about the act of suicide; grief in one's personal life; uncomfortable emotions; and lack of knowledge.

Regardless of their personal feelings about the moral acceptability of assisted dying, professional nurses have a responsibility to skillfully respond to a patient's request for assisted dying in a compassionate, sensitive way. The patient advocacy role of nursing is central to that response, as is the adage to never abandon the patient. Table 2.1 summarizes the guidelines that professional organizations offer to assist nurses in formulating responses to requests for assisted dying.

The Oncology Nursing Society[22] has emphasized that requests for hastening death prompt a frank discussion of the rationale for the request, a thorough and nonjudgmental multidisciplinary assessment of the patient's unmet needs, and intensive intervention for previously unrecognized or unmet needs (p. 1).

Box 2.1 outlines the American Academy of Hospice and Palliative Medicine guidelines for exploring a request for assisted dying.[8] For nurses who practice in Oregon, the Oregon Nurses Association[23] has published detailed guidelines for nurses who choose to be involved in an assisted suicide as well as guidelines for those who choose *not* to be involved but transfer the patient's care to another colleague. In either case, nurses may *not* inject or administer medication intended to end life; subject the patient, family, or other healthcare team members to judgmental comments or actions; or refuse to provide comfort and safety measures to the patient.

# Are There Alternatives to Assisted Dying?

The wish for a peaceful, comfortable death is not unreasonable. Given that assisted dying is not a viable moral or legal option for many individuals, what are the alternatives that could fulfill a desire to control the circumstances of the dying process?

The obvious answer is universal access to expert palliative care. Indeed, there is strong moral consensus among healthcare providers that untreated suffering must never be a justification for assisted dying. However, there are legally and ethically sanctioned options other than assisted dying that may be palatable for some individuals. Refusal of medical treatment is a widely respected means for allowing the dying process to unfold unimpeded by

### Box 2.1 Approaches to Exploring a Request for Physician-Assisted Death: Guidelines from the American Academy of Hospice and Palliative Medicine

- **Determine the nature of the request**

  Is the patient seeking assistance right now? Is the patient seriously exploring the clinician's openness to the possibility of a hastened death in the future? Or is the patient simply airing vague thoughts about ending life?

- **Clarify the causes of intractable suffering**

  Is there severe pain or another unrelieved physical symptom? Is the distress mainly emotional or spiritual? Does the patient feel like a burden? Has the patient grown tired of a prolonged dying?

- **Evaluate the patient's decision-making capacity**

  Does the patient have cognitive impairment that would affect his or her judgment? Does the patient's request seem rational and proportionate to the clinical situation? Is the patient's request consistent with his or her past values?

- **Explore emotional factors**

  Do feelings of depression, worthlessness, excessive guilt, or fear substantially interfere with the patient's judgment?

**Initial responses to requests for hastened death can include the following:**

- Respond empathically to the patient's emotions.
- Intensify treatment of pain and other physical symptoms.
- Identify and treat depression, anxiety, and spiritual suffering when present.
- Consult with specialists in palliative care and hospice.
- Consult with experts in spiritual or psychological suffering or other specialty areas depending on the patient's circumstances.
- Use a caring and understanding approach to encourage dialogue and trust and to ensure the best chance of relieving distress.
- Commit to the patient to work toward a mutually acceptable solution for his or her suffering.

When unacceptable suffering persists, despite thorough evaluation, exploration, and provision of standard palliative care interventions as outlined previously, a search for common ground is essential. In these situations, the benefits and burdens of the following alternatives should be considered:

- Discontinuation of potentially life-prolonging treatments, including corticosteroids, insulin, dialysis, oxygen, or artificial hydration and nutrition
- Voluntary cessation of eating and drinking as an acceptable strategy for the patient, family, and treating practitioners
- Palliative sedation, even potentially to unconsciousness, if suffering is intractable and of sufficient severity

*Source*: American Academy of Hospice and Palliative Medicine (2007), American Academy of Hospice and Palliative Medicine. *Physician-Assisted Death*. 2007. http://aahpm.org/positions/palliatve-sedation. Accessed September 7, 2015,

treatments that will not fulfill the patient's personal goals for the end-of-life experience. Refusal may be in the form of withholding or withdrawing a life-sustaining treatment.

The individual who is not dependent on medical interventions to sustain life and wishes to control the timing of his or her death is faced with a more perplexing challenge. *Voluntary refusal of food and fluids (VSED)* has been identified as a possible option. Although such action requires no direct participation by the healthcare team, nurses can support patients who choose this option by ensuring optimal comfort measures and family support. Depending on the patient's underlying condition, death usually occurs within 1 to 3 weeks.[47]

To evaluate the quality of death associated with VSED, Ganzini and associates[48] surveyed hospice nurses who had cared for terminally ill patients who deliberately hastened death by cessation of eating and drinking. Thirty-three percent of their 307 respondents reported that they had cared for such patients. The most common reasons given by patients for this choice were readiness for death, poor quality of life or fear of poor quality of life, belief that continued existence was pointless, and desire to die at home. Most of the patients had either cancer or a neurologic disease; 85% of the patients died within 15 days after ceasing intake of food and fluids.

The nurses were asked to rate the quality of these patients' deaths on a scale from 0 (a very bad death) to 9 (a very good death); the median score for this sample was 8. The authors concluded that, from the perspective of the nurse participants, most of the patients died a good or peaceful death. Notably, no family or patient perspectives were obtained in this study. Future research should focus on evaluating these perspectives.

*Palliative sedation* represents another alternative to assisted dying. Palliative sedation refers to the use of sedative medications to reduce a patient's awareness of symptoms that have not been sufficiently controlled by other therapies.[49] According to the American Academy of Hospice and Palliative Medicine,[49] sedation to the point of unconsciousness should only be used for "the most severe, intractable suffering at the very end of life" (p. 1). The goal of palliative sedation is to relieve suffering, not to cause death. Palliative sedation may be ethically troubling for both family and professional caregivers because some do not differentiate between this practice and euthanasia. Palliative care experts can provide guidance to assist patients, families, and professionals with appropriate use of sedation and to distinguish palliative sedation from hastened death. In addition, some patients may not find this choice acceptable because they view induction of unconsciousness until the time of death as undignified and as prohibiting communication with loved ones in those final days or hours.

In the following Case Study, a hospice nurse describes a patient's plan to commit suicide in the event he developed intolerable pain and dependency on others.[50]

## Case Study 1: When a Hospice Patient Expresses Interest in Suicide

David, a retired stoic businessman, was admitted to hospice with terminal pancreatic cancer. He told me at my first visit that he was going to commit suicide. He did not ask for my opinion or help, but I understood that he was interested in my reaction. For a time, I said nothing and then asked him what would dissuade him. He reiterated his intent after exploring his concerns about pain and dependency. We made a verbal agreement that he would take no action before my next scheduled visit. Together with the physician, we quickly increased and adjusted medications to manage David's symptoms. At each visit, for at least three subsequent visits, the initial contract between David and me was renewed. Gradually, David no longer talked of suicide, and he died with good pain control at home in the presence of his wife.

I believe that the intense focus on David's plan and alternatives to his proposed action gave David the opportunity to explore other avenues. I believe I was able to gain David's trust, which strengthened as we worked together to ensure that his final weeks were relatively pain free and that his ability to make decisions was encouraged and respected to the end. I recall my own anxiety in my first few visits to David and my resolve to remain calm, caring, and determined to help him live out his days in as much comfort and dignity as possible.

This case illustrates the disturbing consequences of a fear of untreated suffering that can occur at the end of life. The patient's discussion of his plans was the prompt for assessment and interventions to address his needs and fears. The nurse upheld professional standards by exploring the patient's concerns in a nonjudgmental manner, immediately initiating actions in consultation with the physician, and building a trusting relationship over time.

## Summary

Although many requests for assisted dying can be resolved by the application of expert palliative care, a small subset of individuals may seek assisted dying despite such care. Nurses are responsible for responding to patient requests in a manner that reflects professional guidelines and a sense of advocacy for patient rights for quality end-of-life care. Regardless of personal values or discomfort with a request for assisted dying, nurses must apply open communication techniques that allow exploration of patients' needs and fears about the final phase of life.

## References

1. World Health Organization. *WHO Definition of Palliative Care*. http://www.who.int/cancer/palliative/definition/en/. Accessed August 18, 2015.

2. American Nurses Association. *Euthanasia, Assisted Suicide, and Aid in Dying*. 2013. http://nursingworld.org/euthanasiaanddying. Accessed August 18, 2015.

3. Mallon J. *Palliative Care: The New Stealth Euthanasia. Celebrate Life*. November-December 2009. http://www.clmagazine.org/article/index/id/OTAwOQ/. Accessed August 18, 2015.

4. Goldstein NE, Cohen LM, Arnold RM, et al. Prevalence of formal accusations of murder and euthanasia against physicians. *J Palliat Med*. 2012;15:334–339.

5. Friend ML. Physician-assisted suicide: death with dignity? *J Nurs Law*. 2011;14:110–116.

6. Jannette J, Bosek MSD, Rambur B. Advanced practice registered nurse intended actions toward patient-directed dying. *JONA Healthc Law Ethics Regul*. 2013;15:80–88.

7. Boudreau JD, Somerville MA. Physician-assisted suicide should not be permitted. *N Engl J Med*. 2013;368:1450–1452.

8. American Academy of Hospice and Palliative Medicine. *Physician-Assisted Death*. 2007. http://AAHPM.org/position/pad. Accessed September 7, 2015.

9. American Society of Health-System Pharmacists. ASHP statement on pharmacist's decision-making on assisted suicide. *Am J Health-Syst Pharm*. 1999;56:1661–1664.

10. American Public Health Association. *Patients' Rights to Self-Determination at the End of Life*. 2008. http://www.apha.org/policies-and-advocacy/public-health-policy-statements/policy-database/2014/07/29/13/28patients-rights-to-self-determination-at-the-end-of-life. Accessed September 7, 2015.

11. Shariff MJ. Assisted death and the slippery slope: finding clarity amid advocacy, convergence, and complexity. *Curr Oncol*. 2012;19:143–154.

12. Andorno R. Nonphysician-assisted suicide in Switzerland. *Camb Q Healthc Ethics*. 2013;22:246–253.

13. Kimsa GK. Death by request in the Netherlands: facts, the legal context and effects on physicians, patients, and families. *Med Health Care Philos*. 2010;13:355–361.

14. Onwuteaka-Philipsen BD, Brinkman-Stoppelenburg A, Penning C, et al. Trends in end-of-life practices before and after enactment of the euthanasia law in the Netherlands from 1990 to 2010: a repeated cross-sectional survey. *Lancet*. 2012;380:908–915.

15. Oregon Public Health Division. *Death With Dignity Act Requirements*. 2006. http://public.health.oregon.gov/ProviderPartnerResources/EvaluationResearch/DeathwithDignityAct/Pages/index.aspx. Accessed August 18, 2015.

16. Tucker KL. In the laboratory of the states: the progress of *Glucksberg's* invitation to states to address end-of-life choices. *Mich Law Rev*. 2008;106:1593–1611.

17. Hedberg K, Tolle S. Putting Oregon's Death With Dignity Act in perspective: characteristics of descendants who did not participate. *J Clin Ethics*. 2009;20:133–135.

18. American Nurses Association. *Registered Nurses' Roles and Responsibilities in Providing Expert Care and Counseling at the End of Life*. 2010.

http://nursingworld.org/MainMenuCategories/EthicsStandards/Ethics-Position-Statements. Accessed August 18, 2015.

19. American Society for Pain Management Nursing. *Position Statement on Assisted Suicide*. http://www.aspmn.org/documents/PainManagement at the EndofLife_August 2013.pdf. Accessed September 7, 2015.

20. Hospice and Palliative Nurses Association. *Legalization of Assisted Suicide*. 2011. http://advancingexpertcare.org/wp-content/uploads/2015/08/Legalization-of-Assisted-Suicide.pdf. Accessed September 7, 2015.

21. Hospice and Palliative Nurses Association. *Role of the Nurse When Hastened Death is Requested*. 2011. https://www.ons.org/advocacy-policy/position/ethics/hastened-death. Accessed September 7, 2015.

22. Oncology Nursing Society. *Position Statement on Nurses' Responsibility to Patients Requesting Assistance in Hastening Death*. 2013. https://www.ons.org/advocacy-policy/position/ethics/hastened-death. Accessed September 7, 2015.

23. Oregon Nurses Association. *Role of the Registered Nurse in Assisted Suicide*. http://c.ymcdn.com/sites/www.oregonrn.org/resource/resmgr/Docs/ONA_AssistedSuicide_2015-06-.pdf. Accessed August 18, 2015.

24. Vermont State Nurses Association (VSNA). *Position Statement on Physician-Assisted Suicide*. Vermont Nurse Connect. 2004;7(1):12.

25. McClure J. Vermont passes law allowing doctor-assisted suicide. May 20, 2013. http://www.reuters.com/assets/print?aid=USBRE94J0QC20130520. Accessed August 18, 2015.

26. Ferrand E, Drefus J, Chastrusse M, et al. Evolution of requests to hasten death among patients managed by palliative care teams in France: a multicentre cross-sectional survey (DemandE). *Eur J Cancer* 2012;48:368–376.

27. Miller M, Mogun H, Azael D, et al. Cancer and the risk of suicide in older Americans. *J Clin Oncol*. 2008;26:4720–4724.

28. Quill T. Suicidal thoughts and actions in cancer patients: the time for exploration is NOW. *J Clin Oncol*. 2008;26:4705–4707.

29. Spencer RJ, Ray A, Pirl WF, Prigerson HG. Clinical correlates of suicidal thoughts in patients with advanced cancer. *Am J Geriatr Psychiatry*. 2012;20:327–336.

30. Walker J, Waters R, Murray G, et al. Better off dead: suicidal thoughts in cancer patients. *J Clin Oncol*. 2008;26:4725–4730.

31. Fang F, Valdimarsdóttir U, Fürst CJ, et al. Suicide among patients with amyotrophic lateral sclerosis. *Brain*. 2008;131:2729–2733.

32. Maessen M, Veldink JH, van den Berg LH, et al. Requests for euthanasia: origin of suffering in ALS, heart failure, and cancer patients. *J Neurol*. 2010;257:1192-1198.

33. Oregon Public Health Division. *Oregon's Death With Dignity Act—2012*. http://public.health.oregon.gov/ProviderPartnerResources/EvaluationResearch/DeathwithDignityAct/Pages/index.aspx. Accessed August 18, 2015.

34. Smith KA, Goy ER, Harvath TA, Ganzini L. Quality of death and dying in patients who request physician-assisted death. *J Palliat Med*. 2011;14:445–450.

35. Ganzini L, Goy ER, Dobscha SK. Oregonians reasons for requesting physician aid in dying. *Arch Intern Med*. 2009;169:489–493.

36. Morrison RS, Meier DE. *America's Care of Serious Illness: A State-by-State Report Card on Access to Palliative Care in Our Nation's Hospitals*. New York, NY: Center to Advance Palliative Care and National Palliative Care Research Center, 2011. http://reportcard.capc.org/pdf/state-by-state-report-card.pdf. Accessed August 18, 2015.

37. Pain and Policies Studies Group. *Achieving Balance in State Pain Policy: A Progress Report Card* (CY2012). 2013. http://www.painpolicy.wisc.edu/sites/www.painpolicy.wisc.edu/files/prc2012.pdf. Accessed August 18, 2015.

38. Zive DM, Schmidt TA. *Pathways to POLST Registry Development: Lessons Learned*. Portland, OR: National POLST Paradigm Task Force, Oregon Health & Science University, 2012. http://www.polst.org/wp-content/uploads/2012/12/POLST-Registry.pdf. Accessed September 7, 2015.

39. Matzo M, Emanuel E. Oncology nurses' practices of assisted suicide and patient-requested euthanasia. *Oncol Nurs Forum*. 1997;24:1725-1732.

40. Ferrell B, Virani R, Grant M, Coyne P, Uman G. Beyond the Supreme Court decision: nursing perspectives on end-of-life care. *Oncol Nurs Forum*. 2000;27:446–455.

41. Harvath TA, Miller LL, Smith KA, et al. Dilemmas encountered by hospice workers when patients wish to hasten death. *J Hosp Palliat Nurs*. 2006;8:200–209.

42. Campbell CS, Cox JC. Hospice-assisted death? A study of Oregon hospices on Death With Dignity. *J Hospice Palliat Med*. 2012;29:227–235.

43. Jablonski A, Clymin J, Jacobson D, Feldt K. The Washington State Death With Dignity Act: a survey of nurses' knowledge and implications for practice part 1. *J Hospice Palliat Nurs*. 2012;14:45–52.

44. Clymin J, Jacobson D, Jablonski A, Feldt KS. Washington State Death With Dignity Act: a survey of nurses' knowledge and implications for practice part 2. *J Hospice Palliat Nurs*. 2012;14:141-148.

45. Van Bruchem-van de Scheur GG, van der Arend A, Abu-Saad H, et al. Euthanasia and assisted suicide in Dutch hospitals: the role of nurses. *J Clin Nurs*. 2008;17:1618-1626.

46. Valente S. Nurses' psychosocial barriers to suicide management. *Nurs Res Pract*. 2011;2011:650765.

47. Schwarz JK. Stopping eating and drinking. *Am J Nurs*. 2009;109(9):52–61.

48. Ganzini L, Goy E, Miller L, et al. Nurses' experiences with hospice patients who refuse food and fluids to hasten death. *N Engl J Med*. 2003;349:359–365.

49. American Academy of Hospice and Palliative Medicine. *Statement on Palliative Sedation*. http://aahpm.org/positions/palliative-sedation. Accessed September 7, 2015.

50. Volker DL. Oncology nurses' experiences with requests for assisted dying from terminally ill cancer patients. Doctoral dissertation, University of Texas at Austin, 1999. *Dissertation Abstracts International*, 61(01), 199B.

# Chapter 3

# Artificial Nutrition and Hydration

Michelle S. Gabriel and Jennifer A. Tschanz

### Key Points

- Food and drink are synonymous with care, comfort, and hope
- Decreased appetite or inability to tolerate or enjoy food and fluids is often a hallmark of the terminal phase of illness and may be a source of distress for patients, families, and caregivers.
- Initiating or withholding artificial nutrition at the end of life are guided by goals of care, evaluation of benefits and burdens, ethical and cultural considerations, and the beliefs and wishes of the patient and family.
- Patients have the right to refuse hydration and nutrition whether parenteral or oral.
- Nurses have an obligation to provide the necessary information and support as they guide patients and families through the decision-making process regarding artificial nutrition and hydration at the end of life.

## Overview of Artificial Nutrition and Hydration

For many people, food and drink are synonymous with care, comfort, and hope. Discussions and decisions regarding initiating or withholding artificial nutrition and hydration (AHN) at the end of life are guided by goals of care, evaluation of benefits and burden, ethical and cultural considerations, and the beliefs and wishes of the patient and family. AHN are medical interventions, and similar to other medical interventions, the patient has the right to refuse it. Nurses caring for patients and families faced with the decision to start, withhold, or withdraw ANH are responsible for providing education regarding benefits and burdens of these interventions so that informed decisions can be made. This is part of delivering quality care with the rest of the team. The purpose of this chapter is to serve as a resource for nurses to support their ability in caring for patients and families faced with the decision to initiate or discontinue ANH.

# Case Study 1: A Patient With Alzheimer's Disease and Progressive Dementia

Mr. C is a 76-year-old man with Alzheimer's disease and progressive dementia who has been living in a nursing home for 5 years. He is admitted to the hospital for the fourth time in 6 months for aspiration pneumonia. His daughter, who lives in the area, has noticed he has become more cachectic in the last 6 months, has a decreased appetite, and recently has needed encouragement to eat. She notes her father has become weaker and less responsive with time and believes her father is getting closer to death. His son, who lives out of state and is seeing his father for the first time in a year, would like to initiate hydration and enteral feedings through a percutaneous endoscopic gastrostomy (PEG) tube. He believes his father just needs a little help to get through this recent infection. Mr. C does not have an advance directive. Both children state that in previous conversations with their father, he verbalized that he "would not want to suffer when the time comes." They are conflicted about how to proceed with their father's care. The nurse is asked to set up a family meeting with the palliative care team to determine how to proceed with his care.

## Context

In the context of providing palliative care, decisions to initiate or withhold and withdraw ANH can be challenging for the patient, the family, and members of the healthcare team. In many cultures, providing food and fluids is synonymous with caring, hope, and comfort.[1] However, decreased appetite or inability to tolerate or enjoy food and fluids is often a hallmark of the terminal phase of an illness. Individuals and their families may ask for ANH to address a variety of situations (e.g., fears of starvation, weight loss, and dehydration). Clinicians may recommend either artificial nutrition or artificial hydration specific to a particular patient's situation.

As with any palliative care intervention, the nurse needs to understand the patient's illness trajectory, as well as the patient and family goals of care. These can be influenced by a person's culture or religion. The nurse also needs to be familiar with the current evidence for ANH in patients with advanced illness because nurses often participate in conversations regarding treatment options and have a critical role in supporting the patient in identifying interventions that best meet their values and goals.

## Artificial Nutrition

Artificial nutrition is a medical intervention to address *malnutrition*, which has been linked to poorer outcomes such as increased mortality, infections and pressure ulcers.[2] Malnutrition occurs when the body does not get the nutrients it needs.[3] Causes of malnutrition include an inadequate diet, mechanical issues with digestion or absorption of nutrients, and specific medical conditions.[4] In patients with advanced chronic disease or terminal illness, specific causes of malnutrition may result from anorexia, cachexia, and physiologic issues. *Anorexia* manifests with a decrease in appetite, which can lead to a loss of fat tissue. The weight loss that results can be reversible depending on the underlying causes. Many patients with advanced illness experience anorexia.[5,6]

*Cancer cachexia* is a multifactorial syndrome in which there is loss of skeletal muscle that cannot be completely reversed by nutritional support, resulting in a negative impact on functional status.[4] Mechanical issues include malignant bowel obstruction and dysphagia.

## Methods of Administration

Artificial nutrition is the delivery of nutrients to an individual that bypasses the oral route. It can be administered enterally or parenterally. Methods to provide enteral nutrition, which accesses the body's gastrointestinal tract, include nasogastric, nasointestinal, percutaneous gastrostomy, PEG, or jejunostomy access, with PEG being the preferred method of access for long-term feeding.[7] Parenteral nutrition, which instills nutrients directly into the circulatory system, can be delivered through a peripheral vein, using peripheral parenteral nutrition (PPN), or through a central line, using total parenteral nutrition (TPN).

## Benefits and Burdens

Although the benefits of artificial nutrition are clearer in patients who are expected to recover, they are not as clear in patients who have advanced chronic illness or who are terminally ill. Artificial nutrition in the palliative care setting does not always have a positive impact.

In amyotrophic lateral sclerosis (ALS), there are guidelines recommending the use and timing of artificial nutrition because malnutrition and weight loss are prognosticators for survival.[8-10] In patients with cancers of the oropharynx or esophagus, artificial nutrition may be appropriate earlier in the disease trajectory, especially when the cause of malnutrition is directly related to the inability to maintain intake because of mechanical blockages and acute treatment effects (e.g., mucositis secondary to chemoradiation).[11]

Patients and families worry about anorexia and think that artificial nutrition can be beneficial to address both physical and psychosocial symptoms.[12,13] Comorbidity, cognitive function, and social function can predict a patient's success with artificial nutrition.[14] This same study found that predictors of the ineffectiveness of artificial nutrition on clinical outcomes can include severe cognitive impairment and frailty.[9]

Although there may be some benefit in certain populations with end-stage disease, enteral and parenteral feedings are interventions with the potential for associated morbidity and increased suffering. Potential complications associated with the administration of artificial nutrition are listed in Table 3.1. Potential additional burdens include complications from tube placement, increased risk for infection or skin excoriation around

### Table 3.1 Potential Complications of Enteral Support

| Complication | Symptom | Cause |
|---|---|---|
| Aspiration | Coughing | Excess residual |
| | Fever | Large-bore tube |
| Diarrhea | Watery stool | Hyperosmotic solution |
| | | Rapid infusion |
| | | Lactose intolerance |
| Constipation | Hard, infrequent stools | Inadequate fluid |
| | | Inadequate fiber |
| Dumping syndrome | Dizziness | High volume |
| | | Hyperosmotic fluids |

the tube, and use of mechanical or pharmacologic restraints to preserve access.[5,15]

## Specific Impacts: What the Literature Tells Us

### Malnutrition, Anorexia, and Cachexia

In many end-stage diseases, weight loss due to malnutrition, anorexia, or cachexia is a common occurrence. In cancer patients with persistent anorexia and cachexia, artificial nutrition has not been shown to reverse the weight loss.[16] In the terminal phase of diseases such as cancer, artificial nutrition for palliative purposes is rarely recommended.[17-19]

### Dysphagia

When a patient has difficulty swallowing, AN may be considered to ensure that the patient receives adequate nutrition or to reduce the risk for aspiration pneumonia. In certain disease states, such as ALS and dementia, it is a matter of when, not if, dysphagia will occur. For ALS patients, the goal for enteral feeding is to improve quality of life (QOL) and the preferred mechanism to deliver artificial nutrition, if indicated, is through a PEG tube.[20] The onset of dysphagia and the resulting weight loss are indications of when to start artificial nutrition in the ALS patient population.[10] Providers may consider initiating enteral feeds to reduce the risk for aspiration pneumonia; however, studies indicate that enteral nutrition does not reduce, and may increase this risk.[15,20]

### Hunger

Families frequently express concern about their loved one experiencing hunger, or fears about their loved one starving at the end of life, yet patients often deny sensations of hunger in the terminal phase. A study looking at the incidence of hunger in a terminally ill population found that the majority of patients (63%) denied hunger on admission and did not report any hunger during the admission. Of the remaining patients, only 3% (one patient) reported hunger throughout the admission; the others complained initially, but the hunger dissipated over time. All of these patients were offered food by mouth as requested, and the small amounts they tolerated satisfied their hunger; none was given artificial nutrition.[6]

In advanced cancer and dementia, hunger is not a symptom often experienced as a result of the disease process.

### Pressure Ulcers

Patients who are malnourished are at increased risk for pressure ulcers. At the end of life, there is no evidence to support the use of artificial nutrition to treat or prevent pressure ulcers.[15,21] One study demonstrated that in patients with dementia, the use of a PEG tube to administer artificial nutrition was associated with an increased risk for developing new stage 2 pressure ulcers and a decreased likelihood that existing pressure ulcers would heal.[22] Possible reasons for this association include increased likelihood of immobility because of the use of restraints that may be used to ensure that feeding tubes are maintained, and potential for diarrhea owing to the composition of the enteral feeds.[22]

### Survival Time

There is no compelling evidence that artificial nutrition increases the survival of patients with end-stage diseases.[15,20] Studies have looked at the impact of enteral feeds in the dementia population and have found no effect on survival time.[15,23] One study found a median survival time after feeding tube insertion of 165 days and a 64% mortality rate, with half of those who died doing so within the first 2 months after insertion.[24] Another study found no impact on survival time of PEG tube insertion or the timing of the insertion.[23] Other studies have shown an increase in survival in specific populations.

One study compared survival time in dementia patients in Japan who used self-feeding oral intake versus home parenteral nutrition or PEG feeding. The groups who used either home parenteral nutrition or PEG feeding survived almost twice as long as those who did not.[25] In this study, patients were not in the end stage of dementia, which may explain the longer survival time. A further study looked at whether dementia was a risk factor for survival after PEG placement and found no difference in survival between patients with dementia and patients without who received a PEG tube.[26] The authors did not include the stage of dementia in their analysis.

### Quality of Life

There have been few studies that specifically measure QOL for patients with end-stage illness receiving artificial nutrition. In a Cochrane review of enteral tube feeding in an older population with advanced dementia, there were no studies reviewed that measured QOL.[15] Another Cochrane review found two studies that did not demonstrate improved QOL in either a population with motor neuron disease or in a population with advanced cancer who received artificial nutrition.[27]

Some studies have shown that patients and families perceive artificial nutrition to have a positive impact on reducing burden from physical and psychosocial symptoms, such as maintaining the fight against the disease, reducing anxiety due to anorexia, and alleviating symptoms.[12,13] Other studies have looked at the use of artificial nutrition and the prevalence of interventions that may negatively affect QOL such as the use of restraints.

In studies looking at patients with dementia receiving tube feeds, artificial nutrition has been correlated with an increased use of restraints, either physical or pharmacologic.[28,29] In one study assessing family member's perceptions of the impact of a feeding tube, only 32.9% of respondents stated that the intervention improved the patient's QOL.[29]

In summary, artificial nutrition has been shown to have a positive impact on survival and nutritional parameters in certain populations, such as earlier in the disease trajectories for ALS or some cancers. However, there is not enough evidence to support a specific recommendation on when or if, in a palliative care population, it is beneficial to use artificial nutrition.[27] The individual patient's condition and the goals of care need to be considered to best determine the benefit of employing artificial nutrition compared with the burdens of the intervention.

## Artificial Hydration

Hydration is an intervention used to address end-of-life situations such as fluid deficits and altered mental status secondary to medication toxicities. Patients with advanced illness experiencing anorexia may also experience a loss of interest in drinking.[5] During the terminal phase, fluid deficits, similar to malnutrition, may result from anorexia, early satiety, nausea and vomiting, bowel obstruction, dysphagia, and cognitive impairment.[30,31] Some patients and families believe that decreased oral intake and the ensuing dehydration cause suffering. Patients and families are concerned dehydration may precipitate symptoms of delirium, confusion, myoclonus, somnolence, fatigue, neuromuscular irritability, restlessness, thirst, hunger, and constipation, especially in the presence of opioids, benzodiazepines and neuroleptics.[5,31] There is limited information regarding the effects of hydration in addressing these symptoms. Many patients with advanced cancer and their caregivers perceive that hydration provides hope and comfort, improves symptoms and QOL, and fulfills a basic human need for water.[1]

Factors to consider regarding artificial hydration include the following:
- Goals of care
- Advance directives
- Where the patient is on the disease trajectory (e.g., acutely ill or in the dying phase)
- Purpose of hydration (hydration can be used for the temporary relief of symptoms of fluid loss, such as nausea, vomiting, diarrhea, and fevers; to decrease fatigue; to improve mental cognition status associated with medication toxicities; and in respect for cultural and familial beliefs.

### Methods of Administration

Various alternative routes to oral administration are available to meet the goals of care and wishes of the patient and family. Standard methods for replacement of fluids, similar to nutrition, can be achieved by the use of enteral feeding tubes and parenteral methods, such as subcutaneous or intravenous infusion.

Intravenous access requires a competent vein. Clinicians may use permanent access devices if they have previously been placed or if ongoing hydration is anticipated.

Hypodermoclysis is the subcutaneous infusion of isotonic solution. It does not require special access devices and can be used in patients who have poor venous access for intravenous placement. The absorption of the subcutaneous fluids has been found to be comparable with absorption of intravenous fluids when administered appropriately.[32] Hypodermoclysis is relatively uncommon in the United States and is more frequently used in Canada and the UK.[30]

Proctoclysis is used to administer water or saline into the gastrointestinal tract through the rectum using a nasogastric tube. Researchers have found proctoclysis to be safe and economical, but there has been cultural and social reluctance to accept this mode of administration.[33]

There is no consensus regarding the volume or type of fluid replacement. Clinicians make choices based on previous experiences and knowledge of the patient's condition and wishes. Some providers allow the individual to have 1L/day despite the fact that it may be inadequate replacement. Risks and burdens must be considered (Table 3.2).

**Benefits and Burdens**

The decision for hydration needs to include an evaluation of goals of care, discussion of the risks and benefits, and timely reevaluation to determine whether targeted symptoms are improving or worsening. Risks for overhydration, as evidenced by worsening fluid retention, signs of increased shortness of breath, increased emotional distress, or change in mental status, must be monitored. Advantages of not providing artificial hydration can include reduced urine output, leading to reduced incontinence and need for catheterization; reduction of gastrointestinal secretions, leading to decreased incidence of vomiting; and decreased respiratory tract secretions, leading to decreased cough and need for suction.[31]

### Table 3.2 Potential Complications of Routes for Artificial Hydration

| IV Peripheral | IV Central | SC Hypodermoclysis |
| --- | --- | --- |
| Pain | Sepsis | Pain |
| Short duration of access | Hemothorax | Infection |
| Infection | Pneumothorax | Third spacing |
| Phlebitis | Central vein thrombosis | Tissue sloughing |
| | Catheter fragment thrombosis | Local bleeding |
| | Air embolus | |
| | Brachial plexus injury | |
| | Arterial laceration | |
| IV, intravenous; SC, subcutaneous. | | |

Factors arguing against initiating hydration include the increased incidence of pulmonary edema, peripheral edema, respiratory tract secretions, cough, and ascites.[31,34,35] In addition, starting intravenous hydration can cause pain, be distressing, restrict mobility, hinder family contact, and increase the use of restraints.[36]

## Specific Impacts

### Dehydration and Fluid Retention

Dehydration can cause unpleasant symptoms, such as confusion and restlessness, in non-terminally ill patients. These problems are common in dying patients. There is limited research regarding the effect of hydration on alleviating dehydration at the end of life. Results can be challenging to interpret because of the ways various studies define and measure dehydration. Findings suggest that providing artificial hydration may or may not affect physical signs and symptoms of dehydration at the end of life.

One study demonstrated no difference in hydration status after 7 days between advanced cancer patients who were given 1,000 mL/day versus 100 mL/day. The same study also scored four dehydration symptoms (fatigue, myoclonus, sedation, and hallucinations) and noted no difference in the sum of the scores after the 7-day hydration trial.[37]

A retrospective chart review study showed that artificial hydration in the last 48 hours of life had no significant impact on symptoms such as agitation, myoclonus, urinary retention, confusion, congestive cardiac failure, respiratory tract secretions, nausea and vomiting, and ascites.[31] The finding suggests there is no benefit of hydration during the terminal phase of illness. Details regarding volume or reasons for initiating hydration were not discussed.

Depending on the volume of hydration administered, hydration may increase the risk for developing fluid retention symptoms. In a study that measured the effect of hydration volume on terminally ill cancer patients with abdominal malignancies, the patients who were in the hydration group who received 1,000 mL or more of artificial hydration per day 1 and 3 weeks before death were found to have less deterioration in dehydration symptoms than the nonhydrated group who received on average less than 1,000 mL over the 3 weeks before death. However, the patients in the hydration group were noted to have increased symptoms of overhydration, such as edema, ascites, and bronchial secretions. No difference was noted between the groups regarding pleural effusion.[35] A greater prevalence of bronchial secretions in the last 48 hours of life was noted in the group that received more than 1,000 mL/day of hydration compared with the group that received less than 1,000 mL/day.[38]

A national guideline for parenteral hydration therapy established in Japan in 2007 encouraged respecting patient and family wishes, advised conducting a comprehensive assessment of patients' QOL, allowed for TPN to be administered if bowel obstruction is present, and recommended that hydration be decreased to less than 1,000 mL per day if fluid retention is present.[39] A study to measure the efficacy of this guideline demonstrated that providing hydration to patients with advanced cancer according to the guideline led to stable measurements in global QOL, discomfort, most physical symptoms, and fluid retention signs.[38]

### Thirst and Dry Mouth

Thirst is thought to be a nonspecific symptom of dehydration. Effective interventions for thirst and dry mouth as an alternative to artificial hydration at the end of life to reduce symptoms include the following:

- Offering sips of fluids, administering ice chips, and providing mouth care[6]
- Specific to dry mouth, an intensive, every-2-hour schedule of mouth care, including hygiene, lip lubrication, and ice chips or popsicles
- Elimination of medications that cause dry mouth, such as tricyclic antidepressants and antihistamines, if not contraindicated
- Increasing saliva through agents such as pilocarpine (Salagen)
- Treating candida infection if present

### Delirium, Confusion, and Agitation

Delirium can be caused by multiple factors including end-organ failure, dehydration, and medications. Symptoms of delirium can be distressful for patients and families.[30,37] In advanced cancer patients, no significant difference in delirium and agitation was noted between patients receiving more hydration and those receiving less hydration.[35,37] If delirium is related to the accumulation of opioids or other medications, increased hydration as well as other measures may help by facilitating the clearance of toxic metabolites.[38,40]

### Myoclonus

Myoclonus, or involuntary contractions of muscles, is commonly associated with chronic opioid use at the end of life. It has also been reported in cancer patients without opioid use who are experiencing decreased oral intake.[30] There is limited and mixed information regarding the effects of hydration on myoclonus depending on patient setting. In one study myoclonus was shown to improve in the intervention group, which received 1,000 mL normal saline over 4 hours for 2 days versus 100 mL.[41] However, no difference in myoclonus symptoms was noted between patients with advanced abdominal malignancies in the hydration group who were given on average 838 to 1405 mL/day during the last 3 weeks of life and patients in the nonhydration group who received on average 200 mL per day.

### Survival Benefit

There is limited research regarding the survival benefit of hydration. Two studies noted that hydration provided no survival benefit for terminally ill cancer patients with short prognosis.[31,37]

### Quality of Life

There is limited research regarding the effect of hydration on QOL in terminally ill patients. Research of patients with advanced cancer shows that parenteral hydration of 1,000 mL per day did not improve symptoms associated with QOL over placebo of 100 mL per day.[37] Another study showed that QOL measurements remained stable when hydration was administered according to Japanese guidelines that took into account QOL and symptoms of fluid retention, whether patients received small (<1,000 mL per day) or large (>1,000 mL per day) volumes of hydration.[38] In summary, parenteral hydration has been found to be effective in temporary, short-term situations to alleviate symptoms related to dehydration and improve mental cognition. In the palliative care setting, research does not support that parenteral hydration improves signs of dehydration, survival, or QOL.[37] In the setting of delirium related to opioid toxicity, there is mixed evidence supporting hydration and possible opioid rotation to improve delirium symptoms. When deciding to initiate or stop hydration, it is important to assess goals of care, risks and benefits, and the patient's preferences.

## Case Study 2: A Patient With Metastatic Breast Cancer to the Brain

Ms. C is a 44-year-old woman with metastatic breast cancer to the brain who was admitted to the inpatient hospice unit because of a change in mental status. Her family did not want her young children to see her "behaving funny" at home. It was felt by providers that she was experiencing delirium associated with a recent increase in her opioid and diuretic medications. The doctor recommended intravenous hydration through her port. After 4 days of hydration and alterations in medication doses, her cognitive status improved—she was alert and returned home.

She was rehospitalized 1 month later because of mental status changes, and at that time progressive disease was noted in her brain, liver, and bones. Her family requested that hydration be restarted because it had worked previously. After 4 days of hydration, her cognitive status did not improve. She was noted to be less responsive to touch and painful stimuli, to have increased labored breathing, and to have edema in her legs. The doctor and nurse discussed their concerns for fluid overload with the family and made recommendations to discontinue hydration treatment. Her family, however, wished to continue her hydration, although agreed to a marked reduction in the amount, in hopes of improving her condition because it had previously worked.

## Review of Position Statements and Guidelines

Many professional organizations have published position statements or guidelines on the use of ANH. Common themes across these documents include the following:

- ANH is an intervention that should be evaluated by the patient, family, and care team in terms of its benefits and burdens.[5,42,43]
- ANH is considered a medical intervention that can be refused, withheld, or withdrawn based on the patient's clinical condition and goals of care.[2,5,21,42]
- Decisions about ANH need to reflect the patient and family's values, beliefs, and culture.[5,42]

### Table 3.3 Disease-Specific Guidelines for Artificial Nutrition and Hydration

| Advanced dementia[21] | Feeding tubes are not recommended. Enhance oral feedings by improving the environment and supporting patient-centered approaches. |
|---|---|
| End-stage cancer[18,19] | Use of nutritional support for terminally ill cancer patients is not usually indicated. |
| Amyotrophic lateral sclerosis[20] | Early insertion of a feeding tube is recommended if enteral feeding is determined to be an appropriate intervention. |

In addition to general position statements regarding ANH, disease specific recommendations are summarized in Table 3.3.

## Making a Decision About Artificial Nutrition and Hydration

Decisions about the initiation or withholding and withdrawing of ANH are complex.[44] In addition to the review of the clinical evidence regarding the efficacy of ANH to improve symptoms and QOL, it is important to consider ethical principles and legal precedents that highlight nurses' role in advocating for the patient as well as responsibilities in respecting patient and family wishes. Also affecting the decision-making process are religious affiliation and cultural background, in regard to food and fluids. The nurse's own religious affiliation and cultural background also may influence his or her personal comfort with the concept of ANH and its role at the end of life.

### Ethical Issues

The three ethical principles that are most relevant in decision making for ANH are autonomy, beneficence, and nonmaleficence (Table 3.4).[44]

- *Autonomy* refers to the patient right to self-determination.[44] Respecting autonomy in decisions about ANH means that a patient or, in case of incapacity and absent an advance directive, the healthcare agent or surrogate has the right to accept or refuse the intervention based on personal values and beliefs.[45]
- *Beneficence* means "to do good" and implies that nurses must act in the interest of the patient.[44] The nurse has a responsibility to engage the patient and family in a conversation about their goals and values and about the likely benefit and burden of the intervention, while respecting the individual's values and goals for care. For example, a patient with end-stage cancer may be experiencing dysphagia yet still find enjoyment in small sips of liquid. Although the risk for aspiration exists in this situation, the nurse can exhibit beneficence by supporting the intake of fluids if the patient understands the associated risks.
- *Nonmaleficence* means "to do no harm" and can be exemplified by not administering treatments that increases the risk for suffering or creating a burden that is greater than any benefit.[44]

### Table 3.4 Artificial Nutrition and Hydration: Examples of Nursing Interventions That Reflect Ethical Principles

| Ethical Principle | Nursing Actions |
|---|---|
| Autonomy—respecting an individual's right to make choices regarding care | Encourage a conversation that provides information on the benefits and burdens of artificial nutrition and hydration (ANH) to empower the patient to make an informed decision. |
| | Focus on patient's preferences, especially when working with family and caregivers. Ask, "Did we do everything to meet the patient's goals?" not, "Did we do everything possible?" |
| Beneficence—"to do good" | Seek to understand the patient's goals and values to understand what "good" means for them. |
| | Provide interventions that match with patient goals. |
| Nonmaleficence—"to do no harm" | Evaluate the potential risks or burdens of ANH to minimize harm, taking into account the patient's values. |

## Legal Precedent

Landmark cases such as the those of Quinlan,[46,47] Cruzan,[48] Barber,[47] and Vacco v. Quill[49] have set the foundation for current decision making regarding ANH within the healthcare system.

## Religious and Cultural Issues

To deliver patient-centered care, nurses must recognize the role that religious or spiritual beliefs and culture, including race and ethnicity, play on patient and family values regarding food and fluids at the end of life. Understanding these factors and encouraging a dialogue about patient values will enable nurses to respect patient autonomy and engage in a dialogue on how to meet the patient's needs regarding nutrition and hydration to maximize beneficence and minimize harm. In reviewing common beliefs of various religious traditions and cultures, it is important to remember that not everyone of a particular faith or a particular culture will have the same beliefs.[44] Major religions have varying beliefs specific to the use of life-sustaining therapies such as ANH at the end of life.[50-55] Even within religions, there can be varying opinions or interpretations of religious law to guide decisions on whether to initiate or withdraw ANH. Table 3.5 summarizes beliefs by selected religious traditions specific to ANH.

Culture also affects patient and family perspectives of ANH.[50] Studies have shown variance associated with race in the use of tube feedings. For example, studies looking at the use of feeding tubes have shown higher use by African Americans than by white Americans.[56] Studies have also shown that African Americans have a stronger preference for more intensive care at the end of life.[56]

In a study of Singaporean Chinese caregivers' attitudes toward feeding, researchers found three major themes: (1) a sense of filial piety, in which duty to one's family may motivate a push for more aggressive interventions even if the patient is at the end of life; (2) the link between providing nutrition and hope; (3) the belief that providing food shows caring for their loved one. Similar themes are common across many cultures.[57]

Although there is not a large body of research on how differing religious and cultural backgrounds influence individual preferences for ANH, there are resources that nurses can access for information useful when initiating a conversation with a patient on this issue. Whether it is through position statements from religious organizations or talking to leaders within a particular faith tradition or ethnic community, nurses can seek to understand how these factors play a role with the patient for whom they are caring.

### Table 3.5 Various Religious Beliefs About Artificial Nutrition and Hydration

| Religious Faith | Beliefs |
|---|---|
| Buddhism[50] | Buddhists believe that all beings suffer. |
| | The main focus at end of life is on spiritual comfort. |
| | There is less focus on extending life through artificial nutrition and hydration (ANH) and other interventions. |
| Catholicism[51,52] | Current position (as of 2011) of the Catholic Church focuses on "life prolongation based on fundamental human dignity." |
| | Some within the Church assert that ANH not considered a medical technology, but an ordinary measure to preserve life. |
| | Others feel that ANH should be evaluated using the proportionate/disproportionate framework (ordinary versus extraordinary) on an individual basis. |
| | Catholic healthcare facilities are obligated to offer food and fluids regardless of disease state |
| | ANH can be considered extraordinary in conditions in which the underlying disease would be the cause of death, not the withholding of ANH. |
| Hinduism[50] | Withholding or withdrawal of ANH at the very end of life is acceptable. |
| | Some Hindus fast to prepare for death. |
| Islam[53] | "Guiding purpose of Islamic law is to protect and preserve religion, life, progeny, intellect, and wealth." |
| | Islamic rules regarding care for terminally ill are based on the principle that one should prevent or avoid injury or harm. |
| | Islamic law permits withdrawal of ANH and allowing the disease to take its natural course. |
| | There can be various beliefs among Muslims, so it is necessary to learn about the patient's values. |
| | "Islamic law states that palliative care should not shorten a patient's life, but futile treatment is not justified." |
| | "Islamic law forbids passively or actively causing death." |
| | Nutritional support is considered basic care and not medical treatment, leading to a duty to feed patients who are no longer able to feed themselves. |
| | Opinions vary among different Islamic communities regarding withdrawing and withholding ANH. |

*(continued)*

### Table 3.5 (Continued)

| Religious Faith | Beliefs |
|---|---|
| Judaism[50,54,55] | Provision of food and fluids are considered ordinary measures, not extraordinary |
| | Withholding food and fluids is not consistent with Jewish law |
| | Administration of food and fluids, even via IV or feeding tube, is not considered to be artificially administered |
| | "The religious authorities hold that (ANH) are ordinary supportive measures rather than heroic"[54] |
| | "Terminal dehydration, hospice without provision of ANH, and withdrawing or withholding ANH is not considered aligned with Jewish teaching unless there is proof of 'goses' (less than 72 hours until death) and futility of intervention under any denomination of Judaism |
| | "While the [Israeli] law respects the right of a competent dying patient to refuse nutrition and hydration, it introduces a legal requirement to persuade 'the use of oxygen, nutrition and hydration,' even by artificial means."[55] |
| Protestant[50] | There is diversity in positions regarding ANH across denominations |
| | Common belief that interventions such as ANH that allow time for repentance may outweigh other burdens of treatment |

## Engaging in Conversations About Artificial Nutrition and Hydration

Ethics, religion, and culture, factors that may influence an individual's values specific to AHN, similarly influence healthcare team members' perspectives on AHN as an intervention at the end of life. In one study it was found that providers' religious beliefs or legal concerns influenced their likelihood of recommending ANH as an intervention.[58] Consequently healthcare providers must be aware of their own biases. The setting of care can also influence the use of ANH. In patients with dementia, studies have shown variability in the prevalence of use of a PEG tube by state and by type of healthcare facility (i.e., acute care hospital vs. long-term care facility).[29,59] Most terminally ill patients in the United States receive intravenous hydration when treated in acute care facilities but almost never in hospice settings.[30,37] In addition knowledge or lack thereof of current evidence on how ANH affects outcomes in the palliative care population and on how ANH may affect a particular patient's QOL and quality of death will affect how a nurse or other health professional engages a patient or family in these discussions.[15,58,59]

## Empowering Patients to Make Informed Choices About Artificial Nutrition and Hydration at the End of Life

Nurses can empower patients and families by educating them about symptoms commonly associated with the dying process, the benefits and burdens of ANH as an intervention to treat these symptoms, and alternate noninvasive approaches that can be used to alleviate such symptoms. Ethics education may be helpful to the nurse to better support patients and families in their decisions.[60] Developing communication skills is also important. Nurses who feel ill equipped to provide appropriate information about AHN at the end of life should seek counsel from available resources, such as the clinical nurse specialist or the palliative care team, and then return to the patient and family with information.[61]

## Implementing the Decision

If the decision is made to initiate ANH in a patient to meet the goals of care, the nurse has a responsibility to continually assess the patient's condition, evaluating the impact of the intervention on symptoms and the patient's responses to treatment. ANH can be offered as a time-limited trial to determine whether the patient experiences any benefits from the intervention compared with burdens. Because ANH is often instituted during an acute event while the patient is in the hospital, nurses have the opportunity to inquire about previous medical history or expressed wishes and promote conversations that look at the bigger picture beyond the acute admission.[62] Nurses can also ensure that wishes are elicited and documented by the healthcare team regarding ANH.

If the decision is made to either withdraw or withhold ANH, the nurse can provide emotional support and assurances that the patient's dignity will be respected with comfort care. If the nurse is unable to support a patient or family's decision regarding ANH for religious or personal reasons, it is the responsibility of the nurse to request a change in assignment and for the healthcare system to ensure that a nurse is comfortable in these situations and can provide patient-centered care when ANH is being withheld or withdrawn.

## Summary

The provision of food and fluids is synonymous with caring across many cultures. When a patient experiences a decreased desire to eat or drink as part of the end stage of illness, the patient and family may struggle and seek interventions to extend life, including AHN.

Nurses, with knowledge on the benefits and burdens of this medical intervention at end of life can help frame this information for the patient and family within their particular context, goals, and values and so help guide them. Decisions about ANH are complex and guided by the ethical principles of autonomy, beneficence, and nonmaleficence.[44,45]

## References

1. Cohen MZ, Torres-Vigil I, Burbach BE, de la Rosa A, Bruera E. The meaning of parenteral hydration to family caregivers and patients with advanced cancer receiving hospice care. *J Pain Symptom Manage.* 2012;43(5):855–865.

2. Sobotka L, Schneider SM, Berner YN, et al. ESPEN guidelines on parenteral nutrition: geriatrics. *Clin Nutr.* 2009;28(4):461–466.

3. Zieve D, Eltz DR. *Malnutrition.* http://www.nlm.nih.gov/medlineplus/ency/article/000404.htm. June 14, 2011. Accessed August 18, 2015.

4. Fearon K, Strasser F, Anker SD, et al. Definition and classification of cancer cachexia: an international consensus. *Lancet Oncol.* 2011;12(5):489–495.

5. Hospice and Palliative Nurses Association. Artificial nutrition and hydration in advanced illness. *J Hosp Palliat Nurs.* 2012;14(3):173–176.

6. McCann RM, Hall WJ, Groth-Juncker A. Comfort care for terminally ill patients: the appropriate use of nutrition and hydration. *JAMA.* 1994;272(16):1263-1266.

7. Salva A, Coll-Planas L, Bruce S, et al. Nutritional assessment of residents in long-term care facilities (LTCFs): recommendations of the task force on nutrition and ageing of the IAGG European region and the IANA. *J Nutr Health Aging.* 2009;13(6):475–483.

8. Oliveira AS, Pereira RD. Amyotrophic lateral sclerosis (ALS): three letters that change the people's life. For ever. *Arq Neuropsiquiatr.* 2009;67(3A):750–782.

9. Morassutti I, Giometto M, Baruffi C, et al. Nutritional intervention for amyotrophic lateral sclerosis. *Minerva Gastroenterol Dietol.* 2012;58(3)253–260.

10. Thibodeaux LS, Gutierrez A. Management of symptoms in amyotrophic lateral sclerosis. *Curr Treat Options Neurol.* 2008;10(2):77–85.

11. Pfister DV, Ang K, Brizel DM, et al. *NCCN Clinical Practice Guidelines in Oncology (NCCN Guidelines®): Head and Neck Cancers (Version 2.2013).* J Natl Compr Canc Netw. 2013 Aug;11(8):917–23.

12. Del Río MI, Shand B, Bonati P, et al. Hydration and nutrition at the end of life: a systematic review of emotional impact, perceptions, and decision-making among patients, family, and health care staff. *Psychooncology.* 2012;21(9):913–921.

13. Orrevall Y, Tishelman C, Permert J, Cederholm T. The use of artificial nutrition among cancer patients enrolled in palliative home care services. *Palliat Med.* 2009;23:556–564.

14. Donini LM, Savina C, Ricciardi LM, et al. Predicting the outcome of artificial nutrition by clinical and functional indices. *Nutrition.* 2009;25(1):11–19.

15. Sampson EL, Candy B, Jones L. Enteral tube feeding for older people with advanced dementia. *Cochrane Database Syst Rev.* 2009;2:CD007209.

16. Payne C, Wiffen PJ, Martin S. Interventions for fatigue and weight loss in adults with advanced progressive illness. *Cochrane Database Syst Rev.* 2012;1:CD008427

17. Grilo A, Santos CA, Fonseca J. Percutaneous endoscopic gastrostomy for nutritional palliation of upper esophageal cancer unsuitable for esophageal stenting. *Arq Gastroenterol.* 2012;49(3):227–231.

18. August DA, Huhmann MB; American Society for Parenteral and Enteral Nutrition Board of Directors. A.S.P.E.N. clinical guidelines: nutrition support therapy during adult anticancer treatment and in hematopoietic cell transplantation. *J Parenter Enteral Nutr.* 2009;33(5):472–500.

19. Levy MH, Back A, Baker JN. *NCCN Clinical Practice Guidelines in Oncology (NCCN Guidelines®): Palliative Care (Version 2.2013).* http://www.oralcancerfoundation.org/treatment/pdf/palliative.pdf. Accessed September 12, 2015.

20. Anderson PM, Abrahams S, Borasio GD, et al. EFNS guidelines on the clinical management of amyotrophic lateral sclerosis (MALS): revised report of an EFNS task force. *Eur J Neurol.* 2012;19(3):360–375.

21. American Geriatrics Society. *Feeding Tubes in Advanced Dementia Position Statement.* http://americangeriatrics.org/files/documents/feeding.tubes.advanced.dementia.pdf. May 2013. Accessed August 18, 2015.

22. Teno JM, Gozalo P, Mitchell SL, et al. Feeding tubes and the prevention or healing of pressure ulcers. *Arch Intern Med.* 2012;172(9):697–701.

23. Teno JM, Gozalo PL, Mitchell SL, et al. Does feeding tube insertion and its timing improve survival? *J Am Geriatr Soc.* 2012;60(10):1918–1921.

24. Kuo S, Rhodes RL, Mitchell SL, Mor V, Teno JM. Natural history of feeding-tube use in nursing home residents with advanced dementia. *J Am Med Dir Assoc.* 2009;10(4):264–270.

25. Shintani S. Efficacy and ethics of artificial nutrition in patients with neurologic impairments in home care. *J Clin Neurosci.* 2013;20(2):220–223.

26. Higaki F, Yokota O, Ohishi M. Factors predictive of survival after percutaneous endoscopic gastrostomy in the elderly: is dementia really a risk factor? *Am J Gastroenterol.* 2008;103(4):1011–1016.

27. Good P, Cavenagh J, Mather M, Ravenscroft P. Medically assisted nutrition for palliative care in adult patients. *Cochrane Database Syst Rev.* 2008;4.

28. Di Giulio P, Toscani F, Villani D, et al. Dying with advanced dementia in long-term care geriatric institutions: a retrospective study. *J Palliat Med.* 2008;11(7):1023–1028.

29. Teno JM, Mitchell SL, Kuo SK, et al. Decision-making and outcomes of feeding tube insertion: a five-state study. *J Am Geriatr Soc.* 2011;59(5):881–886.

30. Dalal S, Del Fabbro E, Bruera E. Is there a role for hydration at the end of life? *Curr Opin Support Palliat Care.* 2009;3(1):72–78.

31. Krishna LK, Poulose JV, Goh C. Artificial hydration at the end of life in an oncology ward in Singapore. *Indian J Palliat Care.* 2010;16(3):168–173.

32. Lybarger EH. Hypodermoclysis in the home and long-term care settings. *J Infus Nurs.* 2009;32(1):40–44.

33. Bruera E, Pruvost M, Schoeller T, Montejo G, Watanabe S. Proctoclysis for hydration of terminally ill cancer patients. *J Pain Symptom Manage.* 1998;15(4):216–219.

34. Morita T, Hyodo I, Yoshimi T, et al. Association between hydration volume and symptoms in terminally ill cancer patients with abdominal malignancies. *Ann Oncol.* 2005;16(4):640–647.

35. Nakajima N, Hata Y, Kusumuto K. A clinical study on the influence of hydration volume on the signs of terminally ill cancer patients with abdominal malignancies. *J Palliat Med.* 2013;16(2):185–189.

36. Fainsinger RL, Bruera E. When to treat dehydration in a terminally ill patient? *Support Care Cancer.* 1997;5(3):205–211.

37. Bruera E, Hui D, Dalal S, et al. Parenteral hydration in patients with advanced cancer: a multicenter, double-blind, placebo-controlled randomized trial. *J Clin Oncol.* 2013;31(1):111–118.

38. Yamaguchi T, Morita T, Shinjo T, et al. Effect of parenteral hydration therapy based on the Japanese national clinical guideline on quality of life, discomfort, and symptom intensity in patients with advanced cancer. *J Pain Symptom Manage.* 2012;43(6):1001–1012.

39. Morita T, Bito S, Koyama H, Uchitomi Y, Adachi I. Development of a national clinical guideline for artificial hydration therapy for terminally ill patients with cancer. *J Palliat Med.* 2007:10(3):770–780.

40. Galanakis G, Mayo NE, Gagnon B. Assessing the role of hydration in delirium at the end of life. *Curr Opin Support Palliat Care.* 2011;5(2):169-173.

41. Bruera E, Sala R, Rico MA, et al. Effects of parenteral hydration in terminally ill cancer patients: a preliminary study. *J Clin Oncol.* 2005:23(10):2366–2371.

42. American Academy of Hospice and Palliative Medicine. *Statement on Artificial Nutrition and Hydration Near the End of Life.* 2013. http://aahpm.org/poitions/anh. Accessed September 12, 2015.

43. American Nurses Association. *Forgoing Nutrition and Hydration.* 2011 http://www.nursingworld.org/MainMenuCategories/EthicsStandards/Ethics-Position-Statements/prtenutr14451.pdf Accessed September 12, 2015.

44. Geppert CM, Andrews MR, Druyan ME. Ethical issues in artificial nutrition and hydration: a review. *J Parenter Enteral Nutr.* 2010;34(1):79–88.

45. Best C. Introducing enteral nutrition support: ethical considerations. *Nurs Stand.* 2010;24(37):41–45.

46. Wikipedia. *Karen Ann Quinlan.* http://en.wikipedia.org/wiki/Karen_ Ann_ Quinlan. June 2, 2013. Accessed August 18, 2015.

47. Nash RR. Palliative care: ethics and the law. In: Berger AM, Shuster JL Jr, Von Roenn JH, eds. *Principles and Practice of Palliative Care and Supportive Oncology.* 4th ed. Philadelphia, PA: Lippincott Williams & Wilkins; 2013:748–760.

48. Wikipedia. *Cruzan v. Director, Missouri Department of Health.* http://en.wikipedia.org/wiki/Nancy_Cruzan. May 20, 2013. Accessed August 18, 2015.

49. Wikipedia. *Vacco v. Quill.* http://en.wikipedia.org/wiki/Vacco_v. Quill. January 22, 2013. Accessed August 18, 2015.

50. Heuberger RA. Artificial nutrition and hydration at the end of life. *J Nutr Elder.* 2010;29(4):347–385.

51. Bradley CT. Roman Catholic doctrine guiding end-of-life care: a summary of the recent discourse. *J Palliat Med.* 2009;12(4):373–377.

52. Brody H, Hermer LD, Scott LD, et al. Artificial nutrition and hydration: the evolution of ethics, evidence, and policy. *J Gen Intern Med.* 2011;26(9):1053–1058.

53. Alsolamy S. Islamic views on artificial nutrition and hydration in terminally ill patients. *Bioethics.* 2012;28(2):96–99.

54. Rosner F, Abramson N. Fluids and nutrition: perspectives from Jewish Law (Halachah). *South Med J.* 2009;102(3):248–250.

55. Ravitsky V. A Jewish perspective on the refusal of life-sustaining therapies: culture as shaping bioethical discourse. *Am J Bioeth.* 2009;9(4):60–62.

56. Modi S, Velde B, Gessert CE. Perspectives of community members regarding tube feeding in patients with end-stage dementia: findings from African-American and Caucasian focus groups. *Omega.* 2010–2011;62(1):77–91.

57. Chai HZ, Radha Krishna LK, Wong VH. Feeding: what it means to patients and caregivers and how these views influence Singaporean Chinese caregivers' decisions to continue feeding at the end of life. *Am J Hosp Palliat Care.* 2014; 31(2):166–71

58. Duke G, Northam S. Discrepancies among physicians regarding knowledge, attitudes, and practices in end-of-life care. *J Hosp Palliat Nurs.* 2009;11(1):52–59.
59. Cardin F. Special considerations for endoscopists on PEG indications in older patients. *ISRN Gastroenterol.* 2012;2012:607149.
60. Monturo C, Hook K. From means to ends: artificial nutrition and hydration. *Nurs Clin North Am.* 2009;44(4):505–515.
61. Mahon MM. Clinical decision making in palliative care and end of life care. *Nurs Clin North Am.* 2010;45(3):345–362.
62. Coyne PJ, Lyckholm LJ. Artificial nutrition for cognitively impaired individuals. *J Hosp Palliat Nurs.* 2010;12(4):263–267.

# Chapter 4

# End-of-Life Care for Patients With Mental Illness and Personality Disorders

Betty D. Morgan

> ### Key Points
> - Enhanced communication skills with an emphasis on therapeutic communication are needed to work with patients with serious mental illness (SMI) and personality disorders (PDs).
> - Ethical issues including capacity and competency may arise when working with people with SMI or PD, but simply having a diagnosis of SMI or PD does not necessarily indicate lack of capacity or competency.
> - Redefinition of family may need to take place to include the patients' support systems in their care.
> - Consultation and collaboration are essential in caring for the population of people with SMI or PD to meet the needs of the patients and their support systems.

Approximately 26.2% of Americans (about one in four) aged 18 years and older are diagnosed with a mental disorder in any given year. This translates to more than 57 million people in the United States. A smaller number of people, approximately 6% of Americans (1 in 17), have a serious mental illness (SMI), such as schizophrenia, bipolar disease, and severe depression.[1] Comorbidity is common; almost half of the people who are diagnosed with a mental disorder meet criteria for a second mental disorder, with mood, anxiety, and addictive disorders being the most common comorbid illnesses.[1] The Global Burden of Disease Study presented data revealing that mental illness accounted for 7.4 % of all disease-adjusted life years that measure disease burden.[2]

People with SMI reportedly die 20 to 25 years earlier than the general population worldwide.[3] The increase in mortality has been associated with both natural and "unnatural" causes of death, with unnatural causes defined as suicide, homicide, and accidental death.[4] Comorbid medical illnesses that are commonly observed in those with SMI include hypertension, cardiac disease, diabetes, and other metabolic conditions, such as respiratory illnesses, obesity, renal disease, cerebrovascular disease, cancer, and HIV/AIDS.[4,5] Additionally, an estimated one-third to one-half of the homeless people in the world have schizophrenia.[6-9]

Sixty percent of premature deaths in persons with schizophrenia are due to medical conditions such as cardiovascular, pulmonary, and infectious diseases.[3] Because these illnesses may be related to lifestyle factors such as tobacco use and obesity, in these instances they can be viewed as preventable.

This chapter examines what is known about palliative care and mentally ill patients, including those with SMI and personality disorders (PDs). Special issues related to communication and treatment are presented as well as strategies for care in this population. Ethical issues, including capacity and competency for decision making as it relates to those with SMI and end-of-life care, are also discussed. Collaboration and consultation between providers is essential in providing end-of-life care for those with SMI.

## Research Related to Serious Mental Illness and End-of-Life Care

Little research has been conducted in end-of-life issues with people with SMI, and those who have SMI have been underserved in terms of palliative care. Barriers to both care and research have been cited as capacity of patients to make end-of-life decisions, provider concerns that end-of-life discussions would be upsetting, and lack of provider training and comfort in conducting discussions about end-of-life care.[9,10] However, Foti demonstrated that a group of community-residing adults with SMI were able to designate treatment preferences for end-of life care in response to scenarios involving end-of-life situations.[11] Participants chose aggressive pain management in a scenario including pain and incurable cancer and were divided in their responses between waiting for a defined period before turning off life support, terminating life support immediately, and keeping the person alive indefinitely for a patient with an irreversible coma. The researchers also provided follow-up with participants who were distressed by the research questions but found that none required crisis intervention or were so distressed that psychiatric decompensation was a risk.[12]

Much of the existing research has focused on identifying the increase in morbidity and mortality in this population and understanding what factors contribute to the increase. Most of these studies were conducted in inpatient psychiatric settings where the sickest patients and those with the most comorbid illnesses may be found. Piatt and colleagues[10] broadened the discussion about the higher death rates among those with SMI by examining a population not restricted to the sickest of patients with SMI. The researchers found that by looking at case files from a community mental health center and examining years of potential life lost (YPLL), people with SMI had a mean/standard deviation of 14.5 YPLL +/- 10.6 compared with the general population YPLL of 10.3 +/- 6.7.[10] This study also revealed that despite the fact that more people with SMI died from unnatural causes such as suicide, accidents, and assaults than the general population, most of the deaths were actually attributed to natural causes. Four specific causes contributed to the increased death for people with SMI: cancer, chronic lower respiratory diseases, dementia, and pneumonia.

## Barriers to Care for Patients With Mental Illness

There are several barriers to consistent medical care for those with a mental illness; these barriers exist in primary care settings and apply to palliative care settings as well. Lack of preventive care or an ongoing relationship with a medical provider is a key issue for people with mental illness. People with SMI often seek care later in the course of the disease, resulting in costly services and complex care needs. Inadequate support systems that are common among those with SMI affect their ability to access medical care and navigate the complex health system. Adherence is a major problem in the treatment of people with SMI, and adherence to medical regimes for this population is compounded by mental health and addictive problems, homelessness, or lack of transportation to get to medical providers. Lack of financial resources may complicate the patient's ability to receive timely care or treatment.

Symptoms of SMI can have profound effects on communication, which can result in problems with development of the therapeutic relationship. In addition, symptoms of SMI can have an impact on reporting of problematic symptoms or the effect of treatment on the symptoms. One study in the Veterans Administration system posited that people with SMI may not be able to tolerate lengthy and difficult life-sustaining treatments and might lack the supportive network that helps people endure such treatment. Therefore patients with SMI may also accept comfort care earlier on than patients who do not have SMI.[6] Finally, stigma affects communication about all aspects of care of the medical illness, including assessment, explanation of treatment options, adherence, and the development of a trusting relationship with the patient.[5,6]

## Serious Mental Illness

Psychotic symptoms may occur as a result of certain medical conditions, substance abuse, schizophrenia, schizoaffective disorder, mania, dementia, and depression. SMI includes illnesses such as schizophrenia and other psychotic disorders, bipolar disease, and severe depression. Treatment issues and special concerns in communication will be discussed as they relate to palliative care.

## Schizophrenia and Other Psychotic Disorders

Schizophrenia affects approximately 1% of the U.S. population. However, it accounts for 40% of mental health facility beds and 9% of all hospital beds.

It is a devastating illness to those who are affected—both the patient and the family of the patient. The symptoms of schizophrenia include what are referred to as positive symptoms (exaggerated or distorted function) and negative symptoms (diminution or loss of normal function). The positive symptoms include delusions, hallucinations, and disorganized and bizarre behavior and speech as well as deterioration of social behavior. The negative symptoms include flattened affect, decreased range and intensity of expression, anhedonia, restricted thought and speech, amotivation, apathy, and difficulty in mental focus and ability to sustain attention.[7,8] Other psychotic disorders, including schizoaffective disorder, delusional disorder, brief psychotic disorder, and shared psychotic disorder (*folie à deux*), share many of the same psychotic symptoms with schizophrenia.[6,7]

Psychotic symptoms may also be due to medications, substances, withdrawal syndromes from substances, and delirium caused by other medical conditions. Such etiologies for the presenting symptoms must always be ruled out before assuming that there is a psychotic disorder present. At the end of life, people with SMI may appear to have a worsening of their condition when the issue may really involve an acute mental status change because of delirium, in addition to their underlying illness.

Some of the more limiting symptoms of psychotic disorders that are of particular concern in palliative care settings are the ability to participate in decision making, perceptual difficulties that can affect sensory integration, concrete thought processes, and difficulty in attention and concentration. The effect of perceptual difficulties has been demonstrated in research related to pain sensation in people with schizophrenia. Patients with schizophrenia may have reduced sensitivity to pain, and this could lead to delays in care or treatment.[13]

### Treatment of Schizophrenia and Other Psychotic Disorders

Treatment is based on symptom management. As in palliative care, there is no curative treatment for serious mental illness, and all treatment can be considered palliative in nature. Pharmacologic and nonpharmacologic interventions are both used to treat psychotic disorders; however, nonpharmacologic interventions may not be effective unless interfering hallucinations or delusions are brought under some degree of control. The patient may then be able to participate in nonpharmacologic interventions.

#### *Pharmacologic Treatment*

Table 4.1 lists first-generation or typical antipsychotics. These medications, developed in the 1950s and 1960s, were very effective in the treatment of the positive symptoms, and some—but not all—of these medications had effect on negative symptoms. The negative side-effect profiles of these medications, including extrapyramidal symptoms (EPS), tardive dyskinesia (TD), and anticholinergic effects, had a profound effect on quality of life and medication adherence.[8,14]

In the 1980s, the second-generation or atypical antipsychotics were developed (Table 4.1). These medications reduced both the positive and

### Table 4.1 Antipsychotic Medications

| First Generation (Typicals) | Second Generation (Atypicals) |
|---|---|
| Chlorpromazine (Thorazine) | Clozapine (Clozaril) |
| Thioridazine (Mellaril) | Risperidone (Risperdal) |
| Perphenazine (Trilafon) | Olanzapine (Zyprexa) |
| Trifluoperazine (Stelazine) | Quetiapine (Seroquel) |
| Fluphenazine (Prolixin) | Ziprasidone (Geodon) |
| Thiothixene (Navane) | Aripiprazole (Abilify) |
| Haloperidol (Haldol) | |
| Loxapine (Loxitane) | |
| Molindone (Moban) | |
| Pimozide (Orap) | |

Source: Adapted from Beebe LH. Schizophrenia. In Perese EF, ed. *Psychiatric Advanced Practice Nursing: A Biopsychosocial Foundation for Practice.* Philadelphia, PA: F. A. Davis; 2012:467-509; and Chan P. Psychopharmacology. In: Fortinash KM, Holoday Worret PA. *Psychiatric Mental Health Nursing.* 4th ed. St. Louis, MO: Mosby; 2008.

negative symptoms associated with schizophrenia, improved cognition, and were useful in treatment for patients who were considered treatment refractory. The side-effect profile of the second-generation drugs showed lower rates of EPS and TD and fewer anticholinergic effects. However, the emergence of metabolic syndrome, including pronounced weight gain, diabetes, hyperlipidemia, and hypercholesterolemia, has resulted in the need for close monitoring of their use in treating psychotic disorders.[14] These medications result in cardiovascular problems and compound the existing higher prevalence of cardiovascular problems in people with schizophrenia.

Pharmacologic treatment of psychotic symptoms in conjunction with palliative care treatment should be closely monitored by consultation with the psychiatric providers. Any change in mental status should be immediately evaluated. Screening for the presence of delirium, which can occur frequently at the end of life, should occur with any change in mental status. It should not be assumed that the psychiatric illness is the cause of a mental status change until a physical cause is ruled out. Several of the typical and atypical antipsychotic medications share common metabolic pathways with opioid analgesics. Inhibition or potentiation of the antipsychotic or the opioid medication is possible; therefore, close monitoring is essential.[14]

*Nonpharmacologic Treatment*
Nonpharmacologic interventions include psychotherapeutic strategies such as supportive psychotherapy, cognitive-behavioral therapy (CBT), group therapy, skills training, and complementary therapies. Collaborative care with psychiatric providers can include additional supportive therapy to assist patients facing a terminal illness. People with SMI face the same end-of-life concerns as patients without mental illness, such as dealing with pain and suffering, fear of what lies ahead, fear of becoming a burden, spiritual concerns, financial concerns, and difficulty "saying goodbye."[15] People with schizophrenia may need additional support and extra time to process

medical information. This extra support is best provided by professionals who already have a relationship with the patient, and the psychiatric providers should be included in discussions of treatment options in the palliative care setting.

## Ethical Issues in Caring for People With Serious Mental Illness at the End of Life

There are several ethical issues related to the care of people with SMI at the end of life that require consideration over and above the consideration given to people without SMI. Care of vulnerable populations such as those with SMI carries a greater obligation for nurses to provide advocacy and protection from violation of the patient's autonomy and right to make decisions about care.

### Right to Refuse Medication

In the 1970s psychiatric patients filed lawsuits related to their rights to refuse medication treatment. Legal decisions in Massachusetts and New York, the states where the most prominent cases were filed, resulted in different approaches to the problem. The Massachusetts decision resulted in the Rogers decision, which decreed that a guardian needed to be appointed for incompetent patients to deal strictly with the psychiatric medication in question and that the final decision would be left to a judge. The concept of substituted judgment—that is, what the person would consent to if they were competent—is how the judge evaluated the question of whether to give the guardian the right to overrule the patient's right to refuse medication.[16] Other states have panels, independent consultants, or psychiatrists make the decision about right to refuse medication. It is important to know the state law about the right to refuse medication so that each nurse can practice within the rules and regulations under which he or she is governed.

### Advance Directives

Advanced directives, in terms of decisions about psychiatric care in a future emergency situation, have been a focus of concern over the past decade. Providing patients with the opportunity to discuss their wishes, in advance, has assisted with the need to have a legal competency hearing to determine a course of treatment. Including a discussion of the patient's wishes for end-of-life care is an area that needs further exploration in psychiatric settings. Research has indicated a low rate of advance directives for either psychiatric care or medical care in patients with SMI.[6,10,17]

### Capacity and Competency

The ability to make decisions about treatment is a cornerstone of good palliative care. Controversy can occur when a person loses the capacity to participate in informed decision making or when a competent person refuses life-sustaining treatments. A general rule is that all competent persons have the right to make their own decisions, even when decisions conflict with what a majority would decide under similar circumstances.[17] When the patient is a person who has schizophrenia or another psychiatric disorder, the ability to make decisions may be compromised by psychotic thought processes. However, having a diagnosis of a mental illness, even one with psychotic features, does not automatically mean that a person is incompetent.[15] When treatment decisions of the patient are questioned by providers and there is no advance directive about treatment wishes, then a psychiatric evaluation must be requested.

Capacity indicates the ability to understand the problem and make decisions. A psychiatric provider makes a "clinical assessment of the patient's capacity to function in certain areas."[17] Competency is a legal term and is decided by a court of law based on the capacity assessment of a psychiatric provider. Competency is usually confined to a specific area or task, such as the ability to make a will, the ability to testify in court, decision-making capacity, or the right to refuse treatment.[17] Applebaum and Grisso outlined four criteria used to determine capacity to consent to treatment[18]:

- Patient expression of a preference
- Ability to understand the illness, the prognosis with and without treatment, and the risks and benefits of the treatment (factual understanding)
- Appreciation of the significance of the facts (significance of the facts)
- Ability to use the information in a rational way to reach a decision in a logical manner (rationality of the thought processes)

Intense pain, depression, delirium, dementia, and psychosis are the most common causes of incompetence.[17] However, the existence of one of these conditions does not necessarily mean that a person is incompetent. Careful assessment of each individual is necessary to determine capacity and competency. Competency is a legal term, but most courts do accept the evaluation of capacity provided by the psychiatric professional. A patient is not deemed competent or incompetent until a court of law rules.

## Aggression and Psychotic Disorders

Patients enter healthcare systems in great distress, and palliative care settings are no exception. When the patient has an SMI, the distress may be even greater than in the general population because people with SMI may have inadequate coping resources and are in a crisis state when dealing with a life-threatening illness. Most often, people become aggressive when they feel threatened in some way. The aggressive behavior may be the result of perceptual problems, such as hallucinations or delusions, and it often masks a lack of self-confidence. Aggressive behavior may be a way to enhance self-esteem by overpowering others.[19,20]

There are some important predictors of aggressive behavior, including impulsivity, hostility, family history of violent or abusive behavior, substance use, and irritability.[19,20] Prevention of aggressive behavior focuses on early recognition of escalating behaviors, such as pacing, nonverbal expressions, yelling, or an angry tone of voice. Allowing the person a chance to talk may defuse the situation. It is important for the nurse to use nonthreatening body language and to communicate with a calm but firm voice while conveying respect for the patient and the patient's feelings. Allowing the patient some choice about the situation is often a way to help the patient gain some control.[19]

## Communication Issues and Psychotic Disorders

The cornerstone of both palliative care and psychiatric care is the importance of communication and the establishment of a trusting, therapeutic relationship between the nurse and the patient. Traditionally, psychiatric providers are not comfortable with medically ill patients, and medical providers are not comfortable with psychiatrically ill patients. Additionally, many people with mental illness are housed in nontraditional settings. Staff of any of these settings, including medical hospital units, palliative care units, or psychiatric units, as well as the homeless shelters, prisons, and nursing homes, may be ill equipped to deal with psychiatric problems in the face of terminal illness. Education of all staff about mental illness and end-of-life care in these settings will result in better care for patients with SMI.[5]

There are additional communication issues and strategies involved when providing palliative care to those with psychotic illnesses. The role of stigma affects all aspects of care and communication. Patients may conceal or not report pain and other symptoms because of fear of the meaning of the symptom, self-blame, guilt, anger, or denial. As mentioned previously, mental status changes should be evaluated for a medical cause of delirium before assuming that altered perceptions or hallucinations are the result of psychotic disorder.

If the patient is delusional or hallucinating, then a safety assessment should be completed and arrangements made to keep the patient safe from self-harm. The content of the hallucinations or delusions can be very important. Any thoughts or hallucinations that the patient expresses concerning the need to die or presence of command hallucinations telling the person to die require immediate psychiatric consultation. Patient safety mechanisms, such as evaluation by emergency services (for outpatient settings) or use of sitters or frequent observation (for inpatient settings) should be instituted until the psychiatric assessment can occur.

Maintaining a calm presence and using a quiet tone of voice, nonthreatening demeanor, and stance are important strategies when dealing with all patients who are psychotic. Decrease of environmental stimuli, such as turning off a radio or television, will decrease distractions and help the patient focus on the immediate medical care. Because the ability to concentrate or pay attention may be affected by the mental illness, detailed explanations may be needed, with additional time allowed for the patient to process the information. Conversations focused on understanding what the patient has processed about the information may need to take place over lengthened periods of time. Patients may also tend to focus on concrete parts of the information, and it can be helpful to provide alternative ways to view the situation if a patient appears to be stuck or focused on one particular aspect of the issue. Occasionally, people with psychotic disorders may become more focused and less psychotic in the face of a life-threatening illness.

Patients with SMI who are actively hallucinating or delusional, as well as those who may be delirious and experiencing altered perceptions, should receive explanations of all physical care to be delivered. Before touching the patient, it is important to let the patient know what is to be done because the patient might misinterpret the touch and react as if being assaulted. Patients with SMI may have a different sense of private space and may also react to violations of personal space.

**Family Issues**

For many people with SMI there are strained, distant, or nonexistent ties with their family of origin. Some of this disconnection may result from years of strain, disappointment, financial burden, and fear caused by threatening behavior. Families of patients with SMI may also have their own mental health issues and may use defensive strategies in dealing with the medical problems, such as denial or anger. Additionally, family members may have been dealing with chronic sorrow related to the mental health issues of the family member, may be overprotective, or may be psychologically fatigued from years of caretaking responsibilities. Careful assessment of family functioning in these situations may be beyond the scope of the hospice and palliative care nurse and may require consultation with psychiatric mental health providers.

When the patient is competent and there is discord in the family, conflict may arise if providers are restricted about the information they can give to the family because of HIPPA concerns or patient refusal for family inclusion in healthcare discussions. A family member who has been the caregiver for the patient for years and is then shut out from information about the medical illness and treatment options may respond with anger and frustration. Family meetings may be of help in these situations; if there has been an involved mental health provider, this person should definitely be included in the meetings; if there has been no mental health provider, then consultation for the patient and family with a mental health provider, before a family meeting, may be useful. Finding out which supportive services, if any, have helped the family in dealing with the mental health issues is vital. Groups such as the National Alliance on Mental Illness (NAMI, www.nami.org) have been a tremendous support to families with a member with a mental illness. NAMI also runs support groups for family members, and families may have established connections with these groups; if so, they should be encouraged to increase their participation in these groups. NAMI groups may not be focused on end-of-life issues but are familiar with many of the ethical and legal aspects of caring for someone with a mental illness and may be more appropriate than a support group for families focused only on end-of-life issues. As with any patient and family, careful assessment will be key in developing the best treatment approach for the individual and family.

Many people with SMI are cared for by the state government, and long-term relationships with psychiatric providers or staff of mental health housing programs may have become a substitute for family. The inclusion of these staff into the palliative care team is essential to ensuring that the treatment will be properly performed and to providing the day-to-day intensive support that may be required for the patient. Similarly to family, staff will also have their own particular needs for support because most psychiatric providers do not have end-of-life care experience or education. Fellow patients with SMI are the other component of family that needs to be considered in palliative care of people with SMI. Occasionally, long-term relationships with other people with SMI are the most significant relationships in the person's life. Special needs for support should be considered for this group of people as well. Although palliative care staff may not be involved in delivering this support, the collaborative partnerships with psychiatric providers should be available for support for this group of people.

## Case Study 1: A Patient With Schizophrenia

JD is a 47-year-old Hispanic man with a long-term diagnosis of schizophrenia who is single and is currently living in a group home for people with SMI. Both of his parents are deceased, and he has had no contact with his siblings for more than 20 years. He has had multiple hospitalizations, has lived in homeless shelters, and has been in prison twice for aggravated assaults and theft. He has been stabilized on clozapine (Clozaril) for the past 8 years and is adherent with his medication regime as long as he is in the group home and is given his medication by staff members. He has a long history of poly substance abuse including alcohol and was diagnosed with pancreatic cancer 5 months ago. He has had increasing amounts of abdominal pain since that time, and the staff at the group home are currently having trouble managing his needs for pain medication.

He is followed by a psychiatric nurse practitioner (NP) at the mental health clinic where he has received care for the last decade. The NP decides to make a home visit (which she has done in the past) so that she can see the patient in his home setting as well as meet with the group home staff. On the visit she finds that his apartment in the house is dirty and that he has not emptied trash, including old food for over a week; his personal hygiene is less than optimum, The staff are uncomfortable with the opioid medication that they are giving him and have concerns about the addictive potential of the medication as well as concerns that other patients may try to steal the medication.

The NP talks with both the staff and the JD about a referral for home hospice care, emphasizing the help this would provide for personal care, homemaker services, and closer attention to pain management. This initial discussion is very upsetting—more so for the staff than JD! JD is clear that he does not have that long to live, he has capacity to make his own decisions, and he voices a clear desire to stay in the group home rather than be transferred to a nursing home for care. The staff are shocked to hear that he may die within 6 months and are initially resistant to the idea of hospice care. In talking more with the staff (many of whom are in their early 20s), the NP finds that none of them has seen someone die and that they are very reluctant to take on this kind of care. The NP contacts the group home director following her visit to find out what the policy of the group home is for caring for someone at the end of life (there is no policy) and to discuss JD's wishes as well as the staff concerns. The group home director agrees to meet with the NP and the staff the following week to discuss JD's care.

The NP establishes contact with the area home hospice organization to find out what services would be available and discusses the care with the primary care physician who has only seen the patient once since the diagnosis of pancreatic cancer. The physician states that the prognosis for JD is 6 months or less and is agreeable to the hospice referral.

At the meeting the following week with the group home staff, several staff members express their hesitation about caring for JD "till he dies" but are willing to learn more about hospice care and pain management for the time being. The psychiatric NP agrees to be involved with more home visits and coordinating care with the hospice nurses as well as providing some support to the group home staff. As time passes, at least one of the group home staff becomes a strong advocate for JD and influences the other staff to continue to care for JD in the group home as his disease progresses. The staff from the hospice provided some educational sessions about pain and addiction that addressed the staff concerns and provided a lock box for the opioid medication to ensure safety.

Five months later, JD has a quiet and peaceful death in his group home surrounded by his fellow housemates and staff members.

This case illustrates several issues of importance:

- Capacity and the ability of patients to make their own decisions should be assumed despite diagnosis, unless there is a clear reason to suspect impaired capacity.
- Regular medical care is needed for patients with SMI.
- Expansion of definition of family is needed—often residential treatment staff are the ones with daily contact and may best know the patient's wishes regarding care.
- Education of group home staff is needed in care of the dying.
- Attention to grief and bereavement of the staff and other group home residents is needed.

## Bipolar Disease

Bipolar disease has a fluctuating course and often results in recurrent episodes of depression, hypomania, or mania. People with bipolar disease frequently discontinue their medication because of unwanted side effects or the feelings associated with hypomania that may result in increased productivity and pleasure. Bipolar disorder is often comorbid with other psychiatric disorders, particularly with alcohol or substance use disorders. People with bipolar disorder have more co-occurring medical conditions—especially cardiovascular disease and other problems related to metabolic syndrome—than those with other chronic mental illnesses.[21] As with psychotic disorders like schizophrenia, the use of second-generation antipsychotic medications as mood stabilizers for those with bipolar disease has increased the risk for diabetes and subsequent cardiovascular disease among people with this diagnosis.[21]

Bipolar and related disorders is a separate and new category in the *Diagnostic and Statistical Manual of Mental Disorders*, fifth edition (DSM-5).[7] In past issues of the DSM, bipolar disorder was included in the mood disorders category along with major depressive disorder. Bipolar I is described as having at least one episode of elevated, expansive mood for at least 1 week, causing impairment in occupational or social functioning. "The manic episode may have been preceded by, and may be followed by, hypomanic or major depressive episodes" (p. 323).[7]

Symptoms of hypomania or mania include inflated self-esteem, grandiosity, decreased need for sleep, pressured speech, flight of ideas, increase in activities, and excessive involvement in pleasurable activities that have a high potential for consequences.[7] Severe mania can present more with symptoms of agitation than euphoria and often includes psychotic episodes as well.

Bipolar II disorder is characterized by at least one current or past hypomanic episode and a current or past major depressive episode.[7] In past years, bipolar II was considered to be a less severe form than bipolar I. This is no longer considered true given the amount of time that people with bipolar II disorder are depressed along with the accompanying social and occupational altered functioning that can occur with this disorder.[7]

## Treatment of Bipolar Disorder

As with any psychiatric illness careful assessment is the first step of any treatment. This is of particular concern in treating mood disorders. Inaccurate assessment of depression in bipolar disorder may result in initiation of an antidepressant medication and precipitate a manic episode. Additionally, people with bipolar disorder are at a higher risk for suicidal ideation than those with any other psychiatric disorder.[22]

### Pharmacologic Treatment

Treatment of bipolar disorder includes mood-stabilizing medications such as lithium and other drugs (Box 4.1). When patients are in a manic state or a severe depression, they may lack decision-making capacity, but they are then often capable of making decisions when they become stable. A psychiatric provider should be a part of the palliative care team and provide close follow-up for people with bipolar disorder. Any medications used in treatment of the underlying medical illness should be reviewed for their potential to induce a manic episode.[14] As with psychotic disorders, there are many psychotherapeutic interventions that are used to treat bipolar disorder, but patients frequently need to be stabilized with medications before these treatments can be used effectively.

Treatment of bipolar disorder in the acute phase of either a depressive episode or a manic episode may include medications in addition to the mood stabilizers indicated in Box 4.1. Use of atypical antipsychotic medication is often necessary for stabilization of a person in an acute manic

### Box 4.1 Treatment of Bipolar Disorder

**Mood Stabilizers**

- Lithium (Eskalith, Lithobid)
- Lithium citrate

**Benzodiazepines**

- Alprazolam (Xanax)
- Chlordiazepoxide (Librium)
- Clonazepam (Klonopin)
- Diazepam (Valium)
- Lorazepam (Ativan)
- Oxazepam (Serax)
- Prazepam (Centrax)

**Anticonvulsants**

- Valproic acid (Depakene, Depakote)
- Lamotrigine (Lamictal)
- Carbamazepine (Tegretol)
- Gabapentin (Neurontin)
- Oxcarbazepine (Trileptal)
- Topiramate (Topamax)
- Tiagabine (Gabatril)

**Calcium Channel Blockers**

- Verapamil (Calan)
- Nifedipine (Adalat, Procardia)
- Nimodipine (Nimotop)

Source: Perese EF. Bipolar disorders. In Perese EF, ed. *Psychiatric Advanced Practice Nursing: A Biopsychosocial Foundation for Practice*. Philadelphia, PA: F. A. Davis; 2012:427–464.

---

episode. Benzodiazepines may also be used to supplement the use of antipsychotics and mood stabilizers. Antidepressants may also be used in treatment of the depressive symptoms along with the mood stabilizers.[22]

*Nonpharmacologic Treatment*

A variety of psychotherapies have been used with bipolar disease; most often therapies are used in conjunction with psychopharmacologic interventions. Interpersonal therapy and CBT are two of the most widely used therapies with this disorder. Provision of patient and family education is essential, as is social and coping skills training.[22]

### Communication Issues and Bipolar Disorder

Communicating with someone during a manic episode can be difficult because patients may be emotionally labile, very talkative (with pressured speech), not be able to stop and listen or concentrate, and they often reject help.[23] Patients can be quite charming and even entertaining during some stages of a manic episode. Staff members need to see these presentations as a part of the illness and not join in grandiose discussions or plans. Patients may need to be gently redirected so that they do not go off on tangents unrelated to the medical issue at hand. They may also need firm but caring limits set on behaviors that might affect others' care, such as wandering into other patients' rooms, becoming inappropriately involved in others' care, and intruding in staff conversations with other patients. Assisting patients in calming behaviors such as sitting quietly with the patient or closing the door to the room to decrease external stimuli are strategies that may be helpful. Inclusion of the psychiatric provider in the team will allow for communication of information about the best approach to take with an individual suffering with bipolar disorder.

Often, one of the first symptoms of a manic episode is the decreased need for sleep. Early reporting of change of sleep habits is important because it is easier to help someone regain stability early in the course of a manic episode. If the patient is beginning to exhibit signs of mania or psychosis, then assessment of safety issues and the potential for suicide must be considered. The importance of early intervention in escalating symptoms and good interteam communication cannot be emphasized enough when caring for someone with bipolar disorder.

## Case Study 2: A Patient With Bipolar Disease

Jill is a 45-year-old white woman suffering with bipolar disease. She has had a very difficult course of her disease, with multiple hospitalizations following suicide attempts. Additionally, she has HIV and a long history of heroin abuse. Her HIV has progressed over the past 12 years, and her viral load has not been suppressed sufficiently by the last four medication regimens. For the past 2 years, she has been followed for supportive therapy by a psychiatric clinical nurse specialist.

Jill lives with her older brother who is the only family member who has remained involved in her life. He has had to act as her guardian for a number of years because of Jill's psychosis during manic episodes as well as her severe depression. The physician discusses options for care with Jill and her brother and suggests a referral for hospice care. Shortly after this meeting, Jill stopped taking all of her medications and was rehospitalized with severe depression and suicidal thoughts. She has recompensated and returned to her brother's home. She now wants to live and is very meticulous in adhering to her psychiatric medication. The psychiatric clinical nurse specialist meets with Jill and her brother and brings up the issue of a hospice referral again.

Jill's brother has been unable to accept the prognosis and does not want to involve hospice services at this point. Jill becomes less able to care for herself over the next month and is eventually admitted to the hospital for severe dehydration and unresponsiveness. She is never discharged from the hospital and dies with her brother at her side a week and a half after the hospital admission. Jill's brother is despondent and blaming himself for not helping her more. The hospital social worker refers Jim to the area mental health center for counseling.

This case highlights several factors that are important in the palliative care of patients with mental illness:

- Some patients with suicidal histories may put suicidal tendencies aside in the face of a terminal illness and fight to live, in a different way than their history would indicate, as long as their quality of life is satisfactory.
- Chronic severe mental illness may have depleted family coping resources.
- The family may be in a crisis as a result of unexpected medical illness in addition to mental illness.

## Personality Disorders and Palliative Care

People with PDs can present major challenges for palliative care providers, partly because of the stigma associated with PDs. Personality traits are enduring patterns of perceiving, relating to, and thinking about the world and how one relates to the world.[7] The enduring patterns of response and behavior deviate from social norms and present in the following areas:

- Cognition (ways of perceiving self, others, events)
- Affectivity (range, intensity, lability, appropriateness)
- Interpersonal functioning
- Impulse control

There is a lack of flexibility and maladaptive behavior that can cause impairment in function and distress for the person.[7]

All humans have vulnerabilities that are accentuated when the person is under stress. Approaching personality traits as vulnerabilities that are accentuated by stress, and therefore result in the use of predictable coping mechanisms, can be a useful way to change stigmatized attitudes toward people with PDs. It is important to identify traits or vulnerabilities and move beyond labels so that treatment can be geared to preparing for the expected response by minimizing maladaptive coping mechanisms and replacing them with more functional coping mechanisms.

PDs are grouped into three clusters based on some descriptive similarities. *Cluster A PDs* include paranoid, schizoid, and schizotypal. People with cluster A disorders often appear odd, eccentric, or paranoid. People with paranoid PD have a pervasive distrust and suspiciousness of others. The person will be reluctant to trust or confide in anyone and may suspect that others are trying to cause him or her harm.[7] The person with schizoid PD has a pervasive pattern of detachment from relationships, even with family.

This person prefers solitary activities, lacks close relationships, and may be emotionally detached or have a flat affect. People with schizotypal PD are uncomfortable with close relationships and have cognitive distortions, including ideas of reference, odd beliefs or magical thinking, unusual perceptions, odd thinking and speech, inappropriate affect, and social anxiety.[7]

*Cluster B PDs* include antisocial PD, borderline PD, histrionic PD, and narcissistic PD. People with this group of PDs often appear dramatic, emotional, or erratic, and it is this cluster that often presents the biggest challenge to healthcare providers.[7] Patients with antisocial PD have a pervasive disregard for, and violation of, the rights of others. They fail to conform to most social norms and can be impulsive, irritable, and aggressive at times. People with borderline PD have a lifelong pattern of instability of interpersonal relationships and self-image and either idealize or devalue others, or they fluctuate between the two views of the same person. People with borderline PD are impulsive in ways that are damaging to themselves and frequently have recurrent suicidal behavior. They have a chronic feeling of emptiness and therefore constantly seek attention and contact with others to fill themselves.[7] People with histrionic PD have a pattern of excessive emotionality and attention seeking and can be inappropriately provocative or sexually seductive. People with these traits are easily influenced by others and often consider relationships to be more intimate than they actually are. People with narcissistic PD need admiration, have a lack empathy for others, and have a sense of entitlement.[7]

*Cluster C PDs* include avoidant PD, dependent PD, and obsessive-compulsive PD. These disorders share anxiety and fear as their major characteristics.[7] The person with avoidant PD is hypersensitive to negative evaluation, has feelings of inadequacy, and is severely restrained in relationships. This person is reluctant to take personal risks or engage in new activities.[7] Someone with dependent PD has an excessive need to be taken care of that exhibits itself by submissive and clinging behavior and fear of separation. People with this PD have difficulty making decisions and need a lot of advice and reassurance from others. They have difficulty expressing disagreement with others because of fear of loss of support.

Finally, obsessive-compulsive PD is evidenced by a preoccupation with orderliness, perfectionism, and control. The person with obsessive-compulsive PD shows perfectionism that interferes with completion of tasks, is inflexible and overly conscientious, may be unable to throw out useless objects, and is miserly toward spending for self and others. This person may be quite rigid and stubborn in thought and behavior.[7]

**Treatment of Personality Disorders**

By description, PDs are enduring patterns and, therefore, are not likely to change rapidly. Current evidence does suggest that people with PDs can be treated, but realistic goals must be established for treatment. Symptom management and specific therapies such as CBT and dialectical behavioral therapy have demonstrated effectiveness with specific PDs.[24] The relationship with a psychiatric provider is a primary tool in the treatment of people with PDs. There is no medication with a U.S. Food and

Drug Administration indication for treatment of personality disorders. Comorbid psychiatric conditions are common with PD, so symptom management of anxiety, depression, and other psychiatric symptoms is important to improve quality of life.[24]

### Communication Issues and Personality Disorders

Some general principles related to communication with patients with PD can be identified. Clear information provided verbally and in writing with repeated discussions about the information can help with distortions and misinterpretation that are common in people with PDs. A calm and nonjudgmental approach is also the cornerstone of good communication in the process of developing a therapeutic relationship with patients. All discussion of suicidal ideation should be taken very seriously, and a thorough psychiatric assessment should be performed, even when repeated threats of suicide occur. The therapeutic alliance may take a long time to develop, but nonetheless the development of this alliance is a goal for treatment. CBT techniques are helpful for people with PD to examine maladaptive ways of viewing their environment. Supportive therapy is useful in helping people with PD adjust to the issues that arise in palliative and end-of-life care.

Obstacles to therapeutic communication that occur with people suffering with PD include issues such as resistance, transference, countertransference, and boundary violations.[20] Resistance is often unconscious and is usually employed to avoid anxiety. Transference also occurs when a patient unconsciously transfers feelings or attitudes from one person in their life onto the healthcare provider.[25] Countertransference is the emotional reaction of the healthcare provider toward the patient, stimulated by the provider's own past feelings toward someone in his or her personal life. Boundary violations occur when the healthcare provider goes beyond the standards of a therapeutic relationship and enters a more social relationship with a patient.

Communication issues with patients suffering with cluster A disorders focus on the establishment of a therapeutic relationship because distrust, suspiciousness, and withdrawal from interpersonal interactions are common. Engaging a nonthreatening approach and allowing the patient to engage with the provider at his or her own speed is very important. The intensity of a one-to-one conversation may be difficult for those with cluster A PD; therefore, focusing conversation on an external issue or task may be a helpful way to lessen the intensity.

Communications with people with cluster B disorders are often the most problematic for healthcare providers. People with these disorders tend to have an increased risk for suicide, violence toward others, and self-mutilating behaviors as well as chronic low self-esteem, ineffective coping, and impaired social interactions.[24] Volatile changes in emotion as well as splitting behaviors are characteristic of borderline PD. Development of a consistent approach will minimize the patient's ability to split staff and minimize the heightened feelings that can arise in caring for this population.

Providers should be alert for their own countertransference reactions toward patients with PD because this is a common issue. Patients with PD can evoke strong reactions from staff that may interfere with delivery of quality care. Staff support in working through these reactions so that care is not affected can be provided through consultative relationships with psychiatric providers. Many psychiatric clinical nurse specialists have experience with staff support groups to handle such issues.

Communication issues with people suffering from cluster C diagnoses also focus on the development of a therapeutic relationship geared toward assisting patients in identifying their fears and anxiety as they relate to palliative care treatment and issues.[25] Helping people identify their anxiety, decrease the maladaptive response to the anxiety, and increase their supportive relationships with others is essential in dealing with people within this cluster diagnosis.

## Case Study 3: A Patient With Colon Cancer

Lorraine is a 44-year-old woman suffering from colon cancer with metastasis to the lung. She has been hospitalized twice in the past 6 months and is now readmitted to the oncology unit. The staff is not pleased to hear about her readmission because she was a management problem on her last admission. She was frequently upset with the night shift nurses and called the patient advocate several times a week to complain about them. She also left the unit frequently and was not available at treatment times. She complained bitterly about one nurse and demanded that someone else care for her when that nurse was assigned to her care. This caused a great deal of dissatisfaction among the nursing staff, and most of the nurses were relieved when she was discharged.

The nurse manager greets Lorraine as she arrives for readmission to the unit and sees how frightened Lorraine appears to be. The nurse manager is able to spend a few minutes with Lorraine, during which time the patient is tearful and exhibiting signs of air hunger. She is able to assist Lorraine in becoming more comfortable and to discuss her plan of care. Lorraine acknowledges that "I really gave the nurses a hard time the last time I was here. . . . I don't want to do that again. . . . I am really scared and I don't want to die! Please don't leave me alone. . . ."

The nurse manager is able to assure Lorraine that staff will be with her and temporarily asks one of the unit volunteers to sit with Lorraine while she discusses the care with the doctor and gets medication orders to manage Lorraine's anxiety and air hunger. She then calls the psychiatric consultation nurse and asks for help in developing a plan of care, and she sets up a meeting with the nursing staff to discuss the plan and their feelings about Lorraine as a patient. She updates the nurses, who are able to relate to the frightened Lorraine in a compassionate way and put the negative feelings from the last hospitalization aside.

This case highlights several factors in the care of people with personality disorders:

- The labeling and stigma associated with personality disorders and "difficult patients" can result in less-than-optimal care unless someone is

able to be a "role model" in terms of providing the best care possible for the patient.
- Each encounter with patients with PD may be quite different.
- Identification of maladaptive coping mechanisms may help staff understand patient behavior and assist them in developing a nonjudgmental approach to the patient.
- Allowing time for staff to vent and examine their reactions and feelings in dealing with patients who make them upset can help nurses improve care for patients with PD.

## Summary

Palliative care providers often feel poorly prepared to deal with people with SMI or PD. Conversely, psychiatric providers feel poorly prepared to deal with medical care and end-of-life care. Collaborative partnerships can enhance the care given to people with SMI who are in need of palliative care services. Care delivery sites need to be examined for the optimal situation to provide both palliative care and treatment in an environment that also is able to provide optimal support and treatment by psychiatric providers. If the patient has a preference for a place to receive end-of-life care, all attempts possible can be made to address this preference. If the patients consider a halfway house or psychiatric unit to be their home, and they desire to die at home, attempts to provide end-of-life care in that setting should be discussed, just as they would be with patients wanting to die in their more traditional homes.

Nurses have often been instrumental in making this kind of care possible in a situation that had not previously involved this level of care. As strong advocates for their patients, nurses have found a way to insert themselves into new arenas of care and have developed new collaborative partnerships for the ultimate benefit of their patients. Collaboration between psychiatric providers and palliative care providers is a new area in which nurses can lead the way to ultimately provide new skills for each other and meaningful end-of-life experiences for people with SMI or PD and their families.

## References

1. http://www.nimh.nih.gov/health/statistics/index.shtml. Accessed September 12, 2015.
2. Murray CJL, Vos T, Lozano R, et al. Disability-adjusted life years (DALYS) for 291 diseases and injuries in 21 regions, 1990-2010: A systematic analysis for the Global Burden of Disease Study 2010. *Lancet*. 2012;380:2197–2223.
3. Parks J, Svendsen D, Singer P, Foti M. 2006. *Morbidity and mortality in people with serious mental illness. National Association of State Mental Health Program Directors (NASMHPD) Medical Directors Council*. Alexandria, VA: NASMHPD; 2006.

4. Chang C, Hayes RD, Broadbent M, et al. All-cause mortality among people with serious mental illness (SMI), substance use disorders, and depressive disorders in southeast London: a cohort study. *BMC Psychiatry.* 2010:10:77.

5. Baker A. Palliative and end-of-life care in the serious and persistently mentally ill population. *J Am Psych Nurses Assoc.* 2005;11(5):298–303.

6. Ganzini L, Socherman R, Duckart J, Shores M. End-of-life care for veterans with schizophrenia and cancer. *Psychiatr Serv.* 2010;61(7):725–728.

7. American Psychiatric Association (APA). *Diagnostic and Statistical Manual of Mental Disorders.* 5th ed. Washington DC: APA, 2013.

8. Beebe LH. Schizophrenia. In: Perese EF, ed. *Psychiatric Advanced Practice Nursing: A Biopsychosocial Foundation for Practice.* Philadelphia, PA: F. A. Davis; 2012:467–509.

9. Roshanaei-Moghaddam B, Katon W. Premature mortality from general medical illness among persons with bipolar disorder: a review. *Psychiatr Serv.* 2009;60:147–156.

10. Piatt EE, Munetz MR, Ritter C. An examination of premature mortality among descendants with serious mental illness and those in the general population. *Psychiatr Serv.* 2010;61(7):663–668.

11. Foti ME. "Do it your way": a demonstration project on end-of-life care for persons with serious mental illness. *J Palliat Med.* 2003;6(4):661–669.

12. Foti ME, Bartels SJ, Van Citters AD, et al. End-of-life treatment preferences of persons with serious mental illness. *Psychiatr Serv.* 2005;56(5):585–591.

13. Kudoh A, Ishihara H, Matsuki A. Current perception thresholds and postoperative pain in schizophrenic patients. *Reg Anesth Pain Med.* 2000;25(5):475–479.

14. Chan P. Psychopharmacology. In: Fortinash KM, Holoday Worret PA, eds. *Psychiatric Mental Health Nursing.* 4th ed. St. Louis, MO: Mosby; 2008.

15. Kuhl D. What dying people want. In: Chochinov HM, Breitbart W, eds. *Handbook of Psychiatry in Palliative Medicine.* 2nd ed. New York, NY: Oxford University Press; 2009.

16. Laben JK, Yorker BC. Legal issues in advanced practice psychiatric nursing. In: Burgess AW, ed. *Advanced Practice Psychiatric Nursing.* Stamford, CT: Appleton & Lange; 1998.

17. Schouten R, Brendel RW. Legal aspects of consultation. In: Stern TA, Fricchione GL, Cassem HNH, et al, eds. *Massachusetts General Hospital Handbook of General Hospital Psychiatry.* 5th ed. Philadelphia, PA: Mosby; 2004:356.

18. Applebaum PS, Grisso T. Assessing patient's capacities to consent to treatment. *N Engl J Med.* 1988;319:1635–1638.

19. American Psychiatric Nursing Association (APNA). Coping with aggressive behavior in patients with schizophrenia: a roundtable discussion. In: *Counseling Points: Enhancing Patient Communication for the Psychiatric Nurse.* Ridgewood, NJ: Delaware Media Group; 2006.

20. Perese EF. Prevention of psychiatric disorders. In Perese EF, ed. *Psychiatric Advanced Practice Nursing: A Biopsychosocial Foundation for Practice.* Philadelphia, PA: F. A. Davis; 2012.

21. Kilbourne AM, Post EP, Nossek A, et al. Improving medical and psychiatric outcomes among individuals with bipolar disorder: a randomized controlled trial. *Psychiatr Serv.* 2008;59(7):760–768.

22. Perese EF. Bipolar disorders. In: Perese EF, ed. *Psychiatric Advanced Practice Nursing: A Biopsychosocial Foundation for Practice*. Philadelphia, PA: F. A. Davis; 2012:427–464.
23. McCasland LA. Providing hospice and palliative care to the seriously and persistently mentally ill. *J Hosp Palliat Nurs*. 2007;9(6):305–313.
24. Perese EF. Personality disorders. In Perese EF, ed. *Psychiatric Advanced Practice Nursing: A Biopsychosocial Foundation for Practice*. Philadelphia, PA: F. A. Davis; 2012:601–638.
25. McDonald SF. Therapeutic communication. In: Fortinash KM, Holoday Worret PA, eds. *Psychiatric Mental Health Nursing*. 4th ed. St. Louis, MO: Mosby; 2008.

# Chapter 5

# Poor, Homeless, and Underserved Populations

Anne Hughes

> ### Key Points
> - Poor people are at risk for a poor quality of living and a poor quality of dying.
> - People whose lives have been filled with physical and emotional deprivation may be suspicious of efforts to engage them in "shared" decision making to limit therapy, regardless of the therapy's burden and limited benefits.
> - Many people who are poor have multiple morbidities and other marginalizing social characteristics.
> - Poor people's interactions with the healthcare system are frequently marked by rejection, shame, and discontinuity of care.

Poverty is inextricably linked to increased morbidity, premature mortality, and limited access to both preventive healthcare and ongoing medical care. Beyond the medical outcomes of poverty, the personal and social costs are substantial and often invisible. People who are poor constitute a *vulnerable population*, a term used in community health to describe social groups at greater risk for adverse health outcomes. The root causes of this vulnerability typically are low socioeconomic status and a lack of access to resources.[1] Vulnerable populations by definition are underserved by the healthcare system in terms of access to and quality of healthcare. Underserved communities for palliative care include not just the poor and those without adequate health insurance but also the unbefriended elderly, non–English-speaking persons, mentally ill, those with dementia, the developmentally delayed, nursing home residents, and persons with limited health literacy.[2] When individuals or groups are denied what is regarded as standard-of-care interventions, moral questions about social justice appropriately must be asked.

The Institute of Medicine's report, which evaluated racial and ethnic disparities in healthcare, failed to address the role of poverty in disparities.[3] However, the role of poverty in contributing to inequalities, independent of race and ethnicity, is difficult to decipher because class and race are often closely intertwined.[4,5] Some believe poverty may be most responsible for disparities in healthcare.[5] In a systematic review of social determinants of death in the United States, the researchers concluded that low education, poverty (at both the individual and community level), racial segregation, limited social support, and income inequality were as likely causes of death as pathophysiologic and behavioral causes.[6] In other words, being poor is as an important cause of mortality as are pathophysiologic and behavioral explanations.

Although much has been written about the state of end-of-life care in the United States, until recently not much has been said about those in our society who live at its margins, such as the urban poor.[7-19] Lewis conducted a systematic review of the barriers to accessing quality palliative care among the poor.[20] Compared with those receiving palliative care who were not economically disadvantaged, the poor had less access to specialty care (often because of transportation), received fewer home visits and hospice service if they lived in high crime areas, and were at higher risk for dying in institutions. Additionally, as a result of limited health literacy, more of the economically disadvantaged received more aggressive medical interventions, had fewer discussions clarifying goals of care, and were challenged negotiating complex care delivery systems.[20]

To be poor and to have a progressive, life-threatening illness presents more challenges than either one of these conditions alone. As Taipale[21] elegantly notes, "Poverty means the opportunities and choices most basic to human development are denied" (p. 54). Consider the following questions: What type of death would a person hope for who doesn't have a home or lives in a room without a phone, a toilet, or kitchen? What are the meanings of life-threatening illness and death when premature death is an all-too-common part of life? What matters at the end of life if most of your life has been spent trying to survive day to day? All of these questions, in part, introduce us to the worlds of the poor who are confronting a life-threatening illness. Physical, psychological, and spiritual deprivation is not all that poor people contend with—deprivation also harms the moral self and the ability both to act and to live autonomously.[22]

The purpose of this chapter is to consider characteristics of the poor as an underserved population that place them at risk when seriously ill and when palliative care is indicated.[9] In particular, this chapter looks at a subset of the poor who are homeless or marginally housed and how this affects both access to and quality of care at the end of life. The economic downturn affecting the United States and the world in recent years increased the numbers of persons "doing without." However, this chapter focuses on persons whose "membership" in this group is more long term and not the result of an identifiable global economic crisis; similarly, this chapter does not address the experiences of persons living in extreme poverty in resource-limited countries around the globe.

The experience of being poor is not singular, nor it is universal; poor persons are as diverse a population as people who are not poor. Case studies are used to illustrate the concepts discussed and to demonstrate the need for more research to guide practice. The cases described were modified to disguise identifying characteristics; the cases are reflective of the author's clinical practice and research in an urban area that is greatly affected by

HIV/AIDS and homelessness.[23] Therefore, these cases are not generalizable to all the poor or even to all the homeless. Poverty is only one social determinant that affects health status and access to resources. Persons with many vulnerabilities (e.g., being poor and a member of a minority community, elderly, or having other medical problems) are at the greatest risk for adverse outcomes at the end of life.[24]

## Epidemiology of Poverty in the United States

More than 46 million Americans (approximately one in seven) are poor.[25] The poverty line established by the federal government is based on annual household income. In 2011, a single adult younger than 65 years was considered poor if his or her income was less than $11,702, and a family of four (with one adult and three children younger than 18 years) was considered poor if their annual income was less than $22,891. Most experts believe the federal definition of poverty underestimates the true prevalence of poverty in the United States. For example, the poverty line (annual household income) does not capture cost-of-living differences across the country nor out-of-pocket medical costs. Table 5.1 lists states in which the poverty level exceeds the national average of almost 15% in 2011.[26]

### Table 5.1 States Whose Poverty Rates Exceeded National Average (14.9%) in 2011

| State | Rate of Poverty (%) |
|---|---|
| Mississippi | 21.2 |
| Louisiana | 20.1 |
| Arkansas | 19.4 |
| Kentucky | 19.3 |
| New Mexico | 19.2 |
| West Virginia | 18.9 |
| Alabama | 18.5 |
| South Carolina | 17.3 |
| Georgia | 17.3 |
| Tennessee | 17.1 |
| District of Columbia | 16.5 |
| Texas | 16.4 |
| North Carolina | 16.2 |
| Oklahoma | 16 |
| Arizona | 15.8 |
| Michigan | 15.8 |
| Ohio | 15.8 |
| New York | 15.7 |

Source: Macartney S, Mykyta L. Poverty and shared households by state: 2011. *Am Commun Surv Briefs*. 2012;ACSBR/11-05.

The faces of the poor in the United States disproportionately include persons of color, children, foreign-born individuals, and single-parent families. African Americans have the highest rates of poverty in the United States (27.4%), followed by Hispanics (26.5%), Asian/Pacific Islanders (12.2%), and white, non-Hispanics (9.9%) according to the U.S. Census Bureau Report for 2011.[25] Children have greater rates of poverty than young and middle-aged adults and the elderly. Almost 48% of children younger than 18 years living in a female-headed household were poor compared with 10.9% of children living with two married parents.[25]

Although poverty is not confined to urban areas, as evident in Table 5.1, which includes many states with large rural populations, nearly 85% of the poor live in or near the more populous metropolitan areas, and 52% of all the poor live in inner (or principal) cities.[25] Most of the poor have access to some type of housing or shelter, even if the basic accommodations (telephone, cooking and refrigeration, heat, water, private toilet, and bathing facilities) are inadequate. However, for a small subset, housing is marginal or unavailable. This subset is the focus of the following discussion.

## Definition and Prevalence of Homelessness

Homelessness is defined in the Stewart B. McKinney Homeless Assistance Act as a condition under which persons "lack fixed, regular and adequate night-time residence" or reside in temporary housing such as shelters and welfare hotels.[27] Calculating the number of Americans who are homeless or marginally housed is extremely difficult. Most cross-sectional studies fail to capture persons transiently homeless—the hidden homeless, or those staying with family members, those living in cars or encampments, and others living in single-room occupancy hotels (SROs), sometimes known as welfare hotels.[28] Many of the poor and, in particular, the chronically homeless avoid contact with social and health services.

According to the National Coalition for the Homeless, on any given night between 440,000 and 840,000 Americans are homeless; as many as 3.5 million Americans experience homelessness in a given year.[27] Persons who are homeless are not members of a homogenous group. Some are street people and chronically homeless, whereas others are homeless because of a financial crisis that put them out of stable housing (this number climbed with the great recession and home foreclosures). Street people may be more reluctant to accept services and may have much higher rates of concurrent substance abuse and mental illness, that is, are dual diagnosed.[29] Homeless persons frequently are veterans, victims of domestic violence, the mentally ill, and substance abusers. Although the rates of mental illness and substance abuse are higher in the homeless than in persons who are stably housed, assuming that all the poor or, for that matter that all homeless, suffer from these problems only contributes to stereotypes that fail to see the person who is before us. Domestic violence, mental illness, and substance abuse are not confined to the poor; although poverty does not cause these problems, poverty may well exacerbate them.

# Health Problems Associated With Homelessness and Poverty

Numerous health problems are associated with homelessness. Many of these problems are related to environmental factors such as exposure to weather conditions, poorly ventilated spaces, unsafe hotels and street conditions, and high-crime neighborhoods, where the poor are forced to live.[30] These health problems (Table 5.2) include malnutrition, lack of access to shelter and bathing facilities, problems related to drug and alcohol use, chronic medical conditions, chronic mental illness, and violence-related injuries.[28] One fourth of the homeless have a major psychiatric illness; about one in three persons who are homeless abuse drugs and alcohol.[31] Drugs and alcohol are often used to self-medicate distressing psychiatric symptoms (e.g., anxiety, depression, post-traumatic stress disorder).

The individual effects of poverty on health status are irrefutable.[32] Consider the case of coronary artery disease (CAD): the link between onset of CAD and low socioeconomic status has been established and is believed to be related to lifestyle factors, such as poor dietary habits, tobacco use, and limited physical activity.[33] Poor cardiac outcomes among the poor may also be related to limited access to standard medical care.[33,34] Persons who are poor, on average, have shorter life expectancies than those whose incomes are higher.[6] A survey of the "hidden homeless" in Canada to identify housing, health, and social needs reported that for many in the sample (aged 15 to 69 years), their first experience of homelessness occurred when they were in their teens.[28] Similar to other studies, most study participants were male, all had addiction problems, one third had experienced violence in the prior 6 months, and about 25% reported avoiding being housed in shelters. The medical problems most often cited were addiction problems, mental illness,

### Table 5.2 Health Problems Common Among the Homelessness

| Causes | Manifestations |
| --- | --- |
| Malnutrition | Dental problems, tuberculosis, wasting |
| Lack of shelter and access to bathing facilities | Skin infections, lice, podiatric problems, hypothermia, tuberculosis, respiratory infections, sleep disorders |
| Drug and alcohol use | Overdose, seizures, delirium, sexually transmitted infections (such as HIV, hepatitis B, hepatitis C), trauma, falls, cirrhosis, heroin nephropathy, esophageal varices |
| Chronic mental illness | Paranoid ideation, antisocial behaviors, psychosis, suicide |
| Chronic medical conditions | Hypertension, arthritis, venous stasis ulcers, cellulitis |
| Violence-related injuries | Assaults, homicides, rape |

dental problems, chronic pain, respiratory conditions, and sleep disorders.[28] Health and social needs identified included access to nutritious food, transportation, money management, addiction and mental health treatment, and healthcare services and providers who were respectful and not stigmatizing or demeaning.[28] Curiously housing was not identified as a priority, perhaps in part because the researchers recruited most subjects from homeless service agencies, which would have attempted to link services with housing.

In urban areas, health-care services for the poor are often provided by public health departments, teaching hospitals, faith communities, and nongovernmental organizations—the so-called safety net providers. These services typically are overburdened and unable to meet the needs of the poor and the growing number of Americans who are uninsured who access them. For many of the poor, the emergency department (ED) has become the primary source of medical care.[12,35]

## Where and How Homeless People Die

Limited data are available regarding the socioeconomic factors, places of death, and immediate causes of death of the homeless.[36] Similar to those who are not poor, most poor people die in institutions. For those who are homeless, dying on the street or in jail is also a fact of life.[37]

In the past, causes of death among the homeless included drug overdose; alcohol-related deaths; hypothermia; accidents such as fires, falls, and pedestrian–motor vehicle accidents; and violent deaths related to homicide and suicide. Researchers in Boston analyzed mortality among the homeless for shifts in patterns from previous reports.[36] Electronic databases of a program that serves the homeless were searched along with the state death registry for causes of death noted on death certificates. For the 6-year study period (2003 to 2008), there were 1,302 deaths among the homeless. Drug overdose was the leading cause of death, with opioids implicated in 81% of the drug-related deaths. Younger homeless persons (25 to 44 years) were most likely to die of drug overdose. Besides opioids, 43% of drug-related deaths occurred in persons who were polysubstance users; alcohol was found in almost one third of all drug overdoses.

Heart disease and cancer (in particular trachea, bronchus, and lung cancer) were also significant causes of death in this population. Compared with matched adults in Massachusetts, the homeless aged 45 to 64 years had a two- to three-fold higher rate of death related to these chronic diseases. Most of the deaths occurred in the hospital (53%) compared with community residence (27%) or nursing home (10%). The demographic profile of the decedents was similar to past reports: male (81%), mean age 51 years (range 19 to 93 years), and white (60%). Compared with prior studies, fewer homeless persons died of HIV disease; instead, drug overdose was the leading cause of mortality, and tobacco contributed to other potentially preventable chronic disease–related deaths.[36]

## Case Study 1: A Patient With Lung Cancer Metastasis to the Central Nervous System

Al was a 70-year-old white Vietnam veteran who was diagnosed with lung cancer after coughing up blood. His initial cancer treatment included surgical resection and chemotherapy. Al wasn't surprised by the diagnosis after smoking for almost 50 years. One year after the lung cancer diagnosis, he experienced numbness on one side of his body. He got on the bus to the emergency department (transferred to a second bus to the hospital), where he was admitted and diagnosed with brain metastasis (not the stroke he feared while riding the bus, calling 911 was "expensive"). Al was estranged from his middle-class family after his mother's death while he was in his late teens. He joined the military and was sent to Vietnam. His difficult background included loss of his mother and family, alcohol abuse, loneliness, and shame about being homeless.[11] When the elevator in his SRO was broken, Al was forced to carry his portable oxygen tank up three flights of stairs to his room. The most difficult impact of his illness was the weakness and 40-pound weight loss that made him feel more vulnerable when he was outside of his SRO in a high-crime neighborhood. Al was concerned that if someone bumped into him, he might fall, and he could not defend himself. He had never felt vulnerable like this before his illness, ". . . cause I've been through a war. Why would I be scared about anything?" Never married, Al approached his illness and dying matter-of-factly; he was grateful that he was not leaving a family behind who might be burdened and yet regretted not having a family. Al died in a residential hospice program less than 3 days after he was transferred from a public hospital where he had received care.

Al's story reminds us that persons who are seriously ill and marginally housed are trying to manage their illness, its treatment demands, and its impact on function while simultaneously struggling with their basic needs, such as negotiating stairs when an elevator is not working in an SRO hotel, using public transportation to get to emergency department or to medical appointments, feeling more vulnerable when frail and navigating high-crime neighborhoods, and internally feeling shame for being homeless. Al, like many who are homeless, used alcohol and tobacco to cope with life's demands. His death from lung cancer occurred days after discharge from the hospital; fortunately for Al, he died in a residential hospice, where we can only hope he finally experienced compassion and community.

## Poverty, Life-Threatening Illness, and Quality of Life

An enormous body of evidence has demonstrated health inequities related to race and ethnicity; indeed, eliminating health disparities is a federal policy priority.[3,35] Understanding the role race and ethnicity play in the end-of-life experience of the urban poor is complex, however, in no small part because, as Crawley observed, race and ethnicity have been conflated with socioeconomic (SES) status.[38] For purposes of this chapter, a more focused review of the literature is presented without attempting to untangle the role of race and ethnicity from SES in explaining the poorer outcomes such as quality of life.

In a systematic review of the incidence, treatment, and mortality related to heart failure and SES, the researchers evaluated 28 studies that met inclusion criteria. The review concluded that disadvantaged persons had increased incidence of heart failure, higher rates of admissions and rehospitalizations, inconsistent use of beta blockers for treatment, and overall higher mortality rates than their comparison groups who were more advantaged.[39]

Solid organ transplantation is standard of care for end-stage organ diseases that would otherwise compromise quality of life and shorten survival. The literature has documented disparities among racial and ethnic minorities related to both access to organs and poorer graft outcomes for those who receive organs.[40,41] Risk factors for poorly functioning kidney grafts match the profile of the urban poor: African American, male, older aged, unmarried, unemployed, low income, living in poor neighborhoods, and living longer geographic distance from a transplantation center.[40] Lacking a kidney transplantation for example, results in a person with end-stage renal disease (ESRD) being required to get to the dialysis center (if poor this usually means on bus or on foot) and endure lengthy, uncomfortable hemodialysis treatments usually three times a week indefinitely. This kidney function replacement therapy surely compromises the quality of life.

Poor people endure a heavier burden of cancer according several reports from the American Cancer Society and other researchers.[42] In a special report on cancer disparities and premature deaths, the American Cancer Society stated categorically that poverty was responsible for cancer disparities and premature cancer deaths regardless of race or ethnicity.[43] Edwards and colleagues used a community-based participatory research design to understand the factors that affect cancer disparities in East and Central Harlem compared with more affluent neighborhoods of New York City.[42] Forty study participants' interviews uncovered a number of themes. Many of those interviewed in Harlem believed information needs were vast and included available community resources, prevention and early detection of cancer, accessing cancer care, and symptom management. Additional themes that affected cancer disparities in their community included unmet support needs that allowed discussion of cancer's impact and ways to cope, secrecy about the diagnosis, mistrust of healthcare systems, and strongly held beliefs of stigma, fear, and fatalism. Generally, poor people encounter substantial barriers to obtaining quality cancer care, present with more advanced disease, experience more pain and suffering, and are more likely to die earlier of cancer than their economically advantaged counterparts.[43] Findings of the impact of poverty on cancer care are summarized in Box 5.1.

Barnoto and colleagues conducted a national telephone and mail survey of community-dwelling Medicare beneficiaries to explore racial and ethnic

> **Box 5.1 Poverty and Cancer**
>
> - Poor people lacking access to quality healthcare are more likely to die of cancer than people who are not poor.
> - Poor people experience greater cancer-related pain and suffering.
> - Poor people facing significant barriers to getting health insurance often do not seek necessary care if they are unable to pay for it.
> - Poor people and their families make extraordinary sacrifices to obtain and pay for care.
> - Poor people lack knowledge of available community resources, lifestyle factors that contribute to poorer health outcomes, warning signs of cancer, symptom management strategies, and how to access follow up cancer care.
> - Psychosocial support of both individual, group, and outreach efforts at the community level are lacking.
> - Mistrust of healthcare professionals, teaching hospitals, and researchers is common and a barrier to health seeking.
> - Fatalism, fear, and stigma about cancer are commonly held beliefs that prevent accessing care.
> - Secrecy about cancer interferes with accessing care that may even be available in nearby community.
> - Cultural barriers between health care professionals and the community may results in services that do not take into account the community needs, including health literacy. Many in impoverished neighborhoods are certain that environmental pollution may contribute to cancer rates.
>
> *Source:* Adapted from Edwards TA, Jandorf L, Freemantle H, et al. Cancer care in East and Central Harlem: community partnership needs assessment. *J Cancer Educ.* 2013;28(1):171-178; and Freeman HP. Poverty, culture and social injustice: determinants of cancer disparities. *CA Cancer J Clin.* 2004;54(2):72–77.

differences regarding preferences for and concerns about end-of-life treatment.[44] The sample of 2,847 adults included 2,105 whites (non-Hispanic), 489 blacks (17.4%), and 113 Hispanics (4%). When most subjects were asked about their preferences if they were diagnosed with terminal illness with less than 1 year to live, the responses were quite similar: to die at home, without life-prolonging medications with adverse effects, and without mechanical ventilation if such treatment extended life by 1 week to 1 month. However, compared with white respondents, minority subjects were more likely to prefer more medical interventions, including dying in the hospital, possible life-extending medications regardless of their side effects, and mechanical ventilation for 1 month or 1 week.[44]

In the ethnographic study, *Dancing With Broken Bones: Portraits of Death and Dying Among Inner City Poor,* Moller[12] poignantly recounts and photographically documents the stories of poor patients followed by an oncology clinic in a Midwest city. His insights about the suffering of the

> **Box 5.2 Insights About the Dying Poor**
>
> - Poverty inflicts substantial harm throughout life.
> - Poverty exacerbates indignity and suffering throughout dying.
> - Patients and families are often mistrustful and angry about the care received.
> - Patients, at the same time, may be grateful for the care received.
> - Spirituality plays an important role in providing strength and resilience when dying.
> - Social isolation increases suffering.
> - Hidden and sometimes unexpected sources of support can emerge from family and community.
> - The emergency department is the front door to healthcare.
> - The organization of medical care is frequently fragmented and lacks continuity.
> - Funerals are important rituals, and their cost creates enormous stress for survivors.
>
> Source: Adapted from Moller DW. *Dancing with broken bones: portraits of death and dying among inner-city poor.* New York, NY: Oxford University Press; 2004.

urban poor are profound: "...the dying poor are the quintessential violators of the American dream; they live in the shame of poverty and with the unpleasantness of dying" (p. 10). Because much of a person's worth in American society is connected with social status indicators such as occupation, income, and home ownership, the poor represent those who have not made it, have not lived up to their potential. Being poor then becomes a matter of personal failure rather than a social problem requiring public policy changes.[45] From his longitudinal qualitative study of poor inner-city patients, their families, and their healthcare providers, Moller drew a number of conclusions, which are listed in Box 5.2. His work can perhaps be summed up by saying that the indignities of being poor in America are only intensified when that person is also dying. Unlike for persons who are not poor, dying is not always feared in the same way because for some persons who are socially or economically disadvantaged, dying may represent freedom from the misery of living.[11]

## Clinical Presentations of Advanced Disease in the Poor

Persons who are poor frequently present with advanced disease in part related to delays in diagnosis, mistrust of healthcare systems, and late discussions of advance directives and end-of-life care options.[46] In addition to the late-stage disease presentation, many have significant comorbidities that affect both the palliation of symptoms and the course and treatment of underlying illnesses. These clinical management issues usually occur within the context of complex psychosocial situations, as Case Study 2 illustrates.

## Case Study 2: A Patient With AIDS-Related Highly Aggressive Non-Hodgkin's Lymphoma

Tiffany was a frail 34-year-old woman living with HIV disease who was intermittently homeless. When she was stably housed, she was followed by a case management program for HIV in former sex workers who had been released from prison, typically incarcerated because of drug charges. With the support of her case manager, Tiffany was able to take antiretroviral (ARV) medications that were delivered prepoured, and despite some minor side effects, her HIV was virologically suppressed. She kept her medical and social service appointments and was able, for the most part, to remain clean, sober, and safe. When her boyfriend, who was suspected of abusing her, showed up, Tiffany would disappear for weeks to months at a time. Eventually, after being off ARV treatment, she would present to the emergency department and would be hospitalized with an infection and in a debilitated state.

After being lost to follow-up for almost a year, Tiffany presented to the emergency department with eye pain, decreased vision, and swelling that inverted her eyelid and partially exposed the globe. Magnetic resonance imaging showed a mass suspicious for malignancy. Tiffany's CD4 count was 17, and her HIV viral load was greater than 300,000. A biopsy confirmed highly aggressive non-Hodgkin's lymphoma (NHL). The medical oncologist recommended systemic chemotherapy, which Tiffany accepted, and the radiation oncologist recommended external-beam radiation therapy. Tiffany tolerated inpatient chemotherapy despite some side effects. She was most embarrassed by the appearance of her face when the tumor enlarged. Besides the body image disturbance, Tiffany reported moderate to severe pain, odynophagia, and anorexia.

In the past, Tiffany was known to sell her opioids for crack and for heroin that she injected intravenously. The case manager, who knows her, is torn by seeing that Tiffany is in pain and emotionally and spiritually suffering with this new diagnosis and yet at the same is worried that if Tiffany is given large amounts of opioids, her boyfriend will reappear and Tiffany will stop treatment. Tiffany only got to her first radiation therapy appointment. She has no consistent primary care provider given her disjointed connection with a public health clinic; her medical care is being comanaged by an oncologist and an HIV physician consultant. Tiffany's wishes about end-of-life care are unknown. The oncology social worker who has been assigned to work with her reports that Tiffany does not want to talk about her cancer diagnosis or prognosis. According to the case manager, other than her parole officer and her boyfriend, Tiffany has no known family or friends involved in her life.

Multiple morbidities, especially those related to drug use and domestic violence, complicate therapeutic engagement, symptom management, and other medical management.[47] As Tiffany's case study illustrates, there are many pressing clinical needs: NHL management, decisions about resumption of ARV therapy in a person with history of nonadherence and likely drug-resistant virus, engaging Tiffany (with the support of her care manager) in advance care planning, her safety given the possibility of domestic violence, her risk for continued drug use, and symptom management in light of her high risk for aberrant use of opioids. In Tiffany's case the latter proved most challenging for her providers. Tiffany was sent home with long-acting morphine for twice-daily dosing, dexamethasone, and as-needed antiemetic. Her providers considered starting Tiffany on methadone for pain, but she refused. Ultimately Tiffany presented with tumor recurrence, was unable to see, and refused further cancer treatment; she had stopped taking her ARVs. Tiffany was hospitalized, started on intravenous opioid infusion, and died in the hospital with her case manager and some volunteers at her bedside. Her boyfriend, who was unreachable, never showed up before she died.

Symptom management is critical to engaging a patient in care, to developing a therapeutic connection, and then to negotiating about how to begin tackling the other issues. In Tiffany's case, however, there are competing factors that influenced providers' willingness to aggressively manage her pain. Persons known to be chemically dependent may be denied treatment for pain because of providers' concerns of aberrant or drug-hoarding behaviors. In recent years, increases in opioid prescriptions has resulted in a commensurate increase in drug overdoses; this trend has resulted in calls by the Centers for Disease Control and Prevention alerting prescribers and the public about the heightened risk.[48]

Will Tiffany take the medication as ordered? Is she likely to try again to sell her opioids for crack or heroin? Will she give her prescribed opioids to her boyfriend? How does one manage the severe pain of a patient with aggressive cancer who has diverted opioids in the past? Who will prescribe and monitor opioid medications? Does the local pharmacy even carry the medications? In one study pharmacies in predominantly nonwhite neighborhoods in New York City were less likely to carry opioids for pain management than were pharmacies in neighborhoods serving predominantly white communities.[49] Poor social conditions, criminal activity, and the threat of violence are significant barriers to effective pain management for persons with life-threatening illnesses.[50] While Tiffany was an inpatient receiving chemotherapy, her opioid access was controlled and her response monitored. However, her nurses at times expressed concern about giving scheduled opioids and about responding to her requests for opioids as needed when Tiffany seemed drowsy and yet was insisting that her pain was poorly controlled. How can the nurse know for sure that a patient is in pain and not merely "drug seeking" or attempting to self-medicate the suffering of her everyday existence? Some questions are philosophical and often cannot be answered clinically or with psychometrically validated measurements.

Fortunately, researchers and clinicians are recognizing the clinical dilemma of treating pain in persons who have cancer and or HIV disease and who also have addiction disorders; and some recommendations have been offered.[51-55]

Beyond accurately diagnosing and treating the specific cause of the pain when possible, and psychologically screening for addiction and the risk for aberrant drug behaviors, Kircher and colleagues[51] advise the following: (1) obtain informed consent for opioid use in those with cancer diagnosis and addiction disorder, (2) specify prescription access in agreements, (3) select medications based on underlying pain mechanism and disease course, and (4) incorporate adjuvants. Other recommendations[52,53] include observing for aberrant behaviors such as injecting oral formulations, selling drugs, or an unexplained deterioration in function; monitoring for concurrent alcohol or illicit drug abuse; requiring mental health and addiction counseling; and promoting the use of complementary therapies such as massage, acupressure, meditation, and support groups. Additionally, the clinician is advised to frequently evaluate the pain management plan the "4 As": analgesia, activity (function), adverse effects, and aberrant behaviors. Given the potential risks, thorough documentation of assessment and interventions is essential for medicolegal reasons. Clinicians are further advised to remember that relapse can be expected, particularly when the person is under increased stress.[51] Such was the case with Tiffany's diagnosis of an aggressive and disfiguring lymphoma.

In addition to these quandaries, for many persons who are poor or lack adequate health insurance, access to treatment is a significant factor that influences symptom management. For example, if an antiemetic prescribed to relieve the recurrent nausea experienced by a poor person with hepatocellular cancer is not covered on the Medicaid formulary, or the person is not eligible for a drug-assistance program, then the range of medications used to manage the nausea is limited. High-tech methods to control symptoms are not an option for the person who lives in a tent encampment. Most poor persons are institutionalized to manage uncontrolled symptoms and to provide both chronic and terminal care that cannot be managed sufficiently on the street or in the shelter.[12] It is hoped that changes in healthcare insurance and healthcare delivery systems with the Affordable Care Act will result in early access to care and improved clinical outcomes for more persons underserved by our current health care system.

The management of symptoms associated with progressive illness is further complicated by end-organ diseases, such as liver or renal disease, that may alter the pharmacokinetics of medications used to palliate symptoms. Clinically significant drug-drug interactions are common with the ARV medications that Tiffany restarted. In the U.S. Department of Health and Human Services guidelines for initiating and modifying ARV therapies, discontinuing ARVs is barely addressed and is not recommended even for patients who are terminally ill and very debilitated.[56] Determining whether a patient is experiencing an adverse drug reaction is not easy when the person has multiple morbidities, has rapidly progressive disease, is malnourished, or may be continuing to use alcohol or other substances. When Tiffany refused to continue taking ARVs, despite being warned about the risk for viral rebound and immune decompensation, her wishes were honored. Her decision was difficult, however, for some her HIV providers.

Comorbidities also affect the healthcare providers' ability to realistically estimate prognosis and the nature of symptoms or problems that might occur down the road. Tiffany lived with HIV disease for years. Before the introduction of antiretroviral therapy and prophylaxis of opportunistic infections in the mid-1990s, in all probability Tiffany would not have survived as long as she did, particularly given her risky life on the street without case management. Charting the dying trajectory for the chronic progressive illness may be conceivable, but superimposing the other illnesses and injuries that the very poor live with and manage creates jagged peaks and valleys in a downward course. How quickly the life-threatening illness will progress becomes a prognostication puzzle; some persons who have been living on the street truly seem to have had nine lives.

On the other hand, despite the prevalence of substance abuse among the poor, lack of attention to self-care activities cannot be assumed in all drug users. Some homeless persons who use drugs manage complex HIV antiretroviral regimens that require scrupulous adherence; they must take into account possible interactions with other medications or illicit drugs as well as the need for routine laboratory monitoring of CD4 counts and HIV viral loads.[57] Race, class, and housing status cannot be used as surrogate predictors of who will abuse drugs and alcohol or who will not adhere to treatment demands.

## Barriers and Challenges Providing Palliative Care

As suggested, there are many barriers (structural or community factors) that limit access to quality palliative care for the urban poor and an equal number of challenges (individual and illness-related factors) that are common among the urban poor with advanced disease.[12]

Barriers that influence the health status of anyone living in an inner city include high rates of violent crime and drug use; marginal or substandard housing; limited public transportation; convenience stores that sell more tobacco and alcohol than fresh fruits and vegetables; environmental pollution; oversubscribed and often charity-dependent community health services, if even available; lack of pharmacies and restricted drug formularies; and lack of insurance or a reliable income source to meet basic needs.[17,49,58]

Challenges to providing palliative care to the urban poor with advanced disease include person-specific or illness-related factors summarized in Table 5.3. Illness-related challenges include the prevalence of serious mental illness, addiction, and post-traumatic stress disorder;

### Table 5.3 Psychosocial Challenges in Providing Palliative Care to the Urban Poor With Serious Illness

| | |
|---|---|
| Illness related | - Prevalence of concurrent mental illness and substance abuse<br>- Decisional incapacity<br>- Presentation with advanced disease<br>- Multiple comorbidities<br>- End-organ diseases altering pharmacodynamics |
| Resource challenges | - Health literacy<br>- Family or friend caregiver availability<br>- Need for designated health proxy or agent in the event of decisional incapacity<br>- Chaotic lives that have little space for day-to-day illness demands<br>- Limited ongoing therapeutic relationships with health or social service providers<br>- Survival or addiction may overshadow illness management<br>- Competing role responsibilities<br>- Functional impairments, geographic distances, and transportation limitation compromise appointment keeping |
| Relationships with healthcare system or providers | - Cultural history of racism, discrimination, or rejection in healthcare system<br>- As a result of disrespectful, rude, or dismissive interactions in past; may present as angry, avoidant, suspicious, or nonadherent with care recommendations<br>- Healthcare providers often have different cultural and ethnic backgrounds and worldviews |
| End-of-life (EOL) preferences | - Reluctance to relinquish aggressive medical management<br>- Different assumptions about optimal EOL care, particularly in communities of color<br>- Lack of advance care planning because life is experienced moment to moment<br>- Tendency to equate goals of care modification with abandonment or continued poor care<br>- Spirituality may be a hidden resource for comfort and in guiding decision making |

Reprinted with permission of Hospice and Palliative Nursing Association Reference; Hughes A. Meeting the palliative care needs of the underserved. In Dahlin CM, Lynch MT, eds. *Core Curriculum for the Advanced Practice Hospice and Palliative Care Registered Nurse,*. 2013, Pittsburgh, PA: Hospice and Palliative Nurses Association; 2013:529–544.

multiple comorbidities, including end-organ and other chronic diseases; and presenting for care with advanced disease that may be less responsive to disease-modifying interventions even were such therapies available. Social resource challenges include fragile support systems, health literacy concerns, need for a healthcare proxy or agent if a family member or friend is not available, and chaotic lives in which survival frequently overshadows illness management. Relationships with healthcare providers and systems may be frayed if existent, and providers may come with quite different worldviews and cultural backgrounds than the person presenting for care. In general, the barriers to providing quality palliative care to this population require community-level or policy interventions, whereas some of the challenges noted require person-centered interventions. Both levels of approaches will be discussed following a review of the evidence base for providing palliative care to the urban poor.

## Evidence-Based Palliative Care for the Urban Poor

The evidence base to guide palliative care for the urban poor is sparse and includes reviews, program evaluations, and research that used both descriptive and clinical trial designs. The reviews were found in textbooks and journal articles.[8,19,59] The program evaluations described shelter-based,[60] home care,[61] palliative care programs, and the impact of hospital-based palliative care consultation services on family satisfaction and do-not-resuscitate (DNR) status.[62,63] Research used in-depth individual and group interviews, survey, and clinical trial approaches. Researchers explored attitudes and beliefs about end-of-life care[13,14,64] and barriers to palliative care among low-income cancer patients,[17] tested methods for promoting advance directive completion among this population using a low-literacy version[65] or other methods,[18] described the experiences of the urban poor with advanced disease who were community dwelling or in a dedicated AIDS nursing home unit,[10,11] and portrayed the hopes and concerns about care at the end of life for inpatients at public hospital with serious illness.[16]

Of the available "evidence" evaluated, only advance care planning using a 5th-grade reading level version or other methods, including one-to-one coaching or self-completion, was of a sufficient quality to support its translation into practice.[18,64,65]

## Clinical Interventions and Community-and Policy-Level Approaches

### Clinical Interventions: Importance of Relationships

Developing trusting therapeutic relationships is at the very heart of all clinical interventions regardless of whether the person is impoverished and marginally housed or has social and financial resources. Therapeutic relationships take on a particular salience with those facing serious illness and death. However, developing trusting relationships with persons who have experienced rejection or abandonment or have felt unwelcomed in healthcare settings requires patience and time—scarce resources in busy clinical settings. Moreover, relationships may be more highly valued and trusted by some groups seeking medical care than data-driven guidelines,[66] increasing their importance for patient-centered, culturally sensitive palliative care.

Multiple qualitative studies of the urban poor with serious illness have demonstrated a desire for therapeutic relationships with healthcare professionals characterized by respect, by "sitting down and listening," and by honesty and consistency.[10,11,16,64,67] When patients and providers come from different life experiences, the most basic principles of therapeutic communication are crucial (Box 5.3). These include addressing the person formally unless given permission to use the familiarity of first names, sitting at eye level when interacting, and appreciating that the palliative care philosophy and principles guiding the care approach may be quite foreign or even suspect as a means of denying care (again) or as an "ethically charged" clinical intervention.[59,66]

Davis and colleagues interviewed homeless chronically ill adults about the case management services they received to stabilize their medical conditions and social situations.[67] Four themes emerged from the interview data: (1) participants described profound isolation before receiving case

---

**Box 5.3 Helpful Suggestions for Engaging a Difficult-to-Engage Client**

- Address anyone older than 40 years of age by the title of Mr. or Ms. Ask permission to be on a first-name basis.
- Do not hesitate to shake hands.
- Be prepared to meet people who are more intelligent, more perceptive, and more wounded than you expect.
- Be tolerant. How would you react if you were in that situation?
- Don't make promises you can't keep.
- Don't take it personally.
- Taking time out helps prevent burnout.
- Get to know the community.
- If you feel you have to save the human race, do it one person at a time.
- Providing material assistance (e.g., clean socks, food, hygiene kits) opens people up.
- Usually the most difficult clients are those most in need. Throw the word *noncompliant* out of your vocabulary.
- Make eye contact. If the person does not like eye contact or becomes agitated, avoid using it.
- Keep in mind that people who live intense lives may not particularly like unasked-for physical contact.
- Don't be afraid to ask "stupid" questions; patients' answers are better than your assumptions.
- Adjust your expectations and accept small victories with satisfaction.

*Source:* Patchell T. *Suggestions for Effective Outreach.* San Francisco, CA: San Francisco Department of Public Health, Homeless Death Prevention Project; 1997.

management services, (2) caring relationships with case managers were key to the program's benefit, (3) case managers assisted participants to navigate medical and social service systems, and (4) participants perceived improved health because of the interpersonal and practical interventions. The title of the study report perhaps says it all: "Because Somebody Cared About It. That's How It Changed Things."[67]

## Assessment Considerations

A comprehensive assessment by a nurse includes a history of the illness, treatment, comorbidities, medication, self-care abilities, symptom management, a physical examination appropriate to the presenting complaint and history, and psychosocial information that may shape end-of-life care options. Obtaining psychosocial information over time, rather than in a single session, is more likely to promote a therapeutic connection and to uncover a richer narrative. Admittedly, appointment follow-up difficulties often justify trying to get as much information as possible during an initial encounter. Although various screening or assessment tools for specific aspects of care are available and are recommended in many practice guidelines, determining when or if to use such standardized instruments needs to occur on a case-by-case basis in a population who may be more hesitant to engage in care and suspicious of how this information may be used.

In addition to illness, treatment, comorbidities, medication, self-care, and symptom-related assessment, psychosocial areas to assess include but are not limited to the following[19]:

- Housing—Where do you usually stay at night?)
- Food—Are there times when you are hungry from not having enough to eat?
- Transportation—How do you get to appointments or to the hospital?
- Income—Are you receiving any income or benefits?
- Preferred communication methods—How can we get in touch with you?
- Caregiver availability—Is there someone you can count on when you need help?
- Use of other resources—Do you have a case manager, peer advocate, sponsor, or patient navigator?
- Literacy—Are you much of a reader? How do you like to get information about your health?
- Spirituality—What role does faith or religion play in your life?
- Cultural identity—What beliefs or practices about health and healing are important for us to incorporate into your care?
- Safety—Do you feel safe where you're staying?
- Coping resources—How have you coped in the past when dealing with challenges?
- Substance use—Have you used alcohol or drugs to cope? If so, what difficulties has their use presented in your life?

In addition to using interpersonal interventions to engage the client in a therapeutic interaction, nurses are often required to become knowledgeable about the availability of and the services provided by community agencies. Are pharmacies available, what are their hours, are they willing to accept telephone orders, and what medications are kept on hand? What supportive services are available, such as food and meal programs, case management services, representative payee programs, supportive housing, and crisis mental health and substance abuse programs? What home health or hospice programs service the community, including any restrictions on services because of concerns related to staff safety? Knowing which agencies or services are involved with a client and communicating with them ensure consistency of approach and continuity of care. Advocacy is often required to access services such as pain management, substance abuse treatment, mental health services, and social services for housing and money management.

In summary, developing therapeutic relationships with the poor and homeless requires expecting that their trust must be earned over time (sometimes a long time) and cannot taken for granted; respecting their humanity, no matter how they look, what they say, and what feelings in us they evoke; appreciating their unique stories as influencing their response to illness and death; and, finally, recognizing and addressing their maladaptive behaviors. Case Study 3 may serve to underscore the importance of relationships and knowing the person over time.

## Case Study 3: A Patient With End-Stage Renal Disease on Dialysis and With Suspected Occult Malignancy

Johnny was a 65-year-old African American man with ESRD managed by hemodialysis treatments three times a week for several years. Johnny was never considered a candidate for kidney transplantation. His other medical problems included hepatitis C and cirrhosis, hypertension, cerebrovascular accident with resulting left hemiparesis, chronic obstructive pulmonary disease, polysubstance abuse, depression, vertebral lytic lesion, and recurrent lower gastrointestinal bleed. He had lived in an SRO until, after repeated hospitalizations, he reluctantly agreed to placement in a long-term care facility. Johnny was a self-described loner; he liked to watch people but avoided social events or groups when invited. His social worker described him as not liking to be hassled and wanting to be left alone. Johnny was raised Baptist and periodically would speak to a minister who came to the facility. He described his faith as important and private.

After a lower gastrointestinal bleed resulted in his needing a transfusion, Johnny declined colonoscopy or other workup. An incidental finding on an x-ray after a noninjurious fall revealed a vertebral lytic lesion, but Johnny declined further workup. He began to refuse transport to the dialysis center despite being told the implications of his refusal. When he developed more symptoms (fatigue, nausea, malaise, mental slowing), he would agree to dialysis; when his condition deteriorated substantially, the dialysis center would send him to the emergency department. This pattern was repeated a few times.

Johnny had been estranged from his family; his mother died in the past year, and he had only recently connected with his brother who lived on the other side of the country where Johnny was born and raised. He was seen by a psychologist who determined that Johnny understood the risks of his refusal of dialysis; the psychologist confirmed that Johnny had decisional capacity and further determined his actions were not passive attempts at suicide. Johnny told the palliative care consultant, "I don't want to die ... but living like this isn't good. I want to be more comfortable. Do everything you can to keep me going but I'm not going to dialysis if I don't feel like it ... yeah ... without dialysis, they tell me I'll die." Johnny was tired of dialysis and the demands of this treatment. At the same time and seemingly contradictory, Johnny was not looking forward to death and wanted everything done to postpone his dying (except for dialysis). Johnny wanted to be kept comfortable, but he finally agreed to a DNR order. He understood that at some point his thinking would be affected by not having dialysis and his family would likely be consulted because he had no formal advance directive. Johnny gave permission for his brother to be contacted and to be advised of his condition. Additionally, Johnny asked to see the minister to read the Bible to him and to pray with him.

After refusing almost 2 weeks of dialysis, Johnny agreed to be dialyzed. Immediately after arriving at the dialysis center, the nephrologist called the paramedics to take Johnny to the emergency department for admission. By that time, Johnny was no longer able to make his own decisions. After consultation between the medical admitting team, the facility staff, and Johnny's brother, the decision was reached to accept Johnny's action (refusal of dialysis after years of treatment) was likely more reflective of his values and wishes than his contradictory remarks about wanting everything done to keep him going, to honor his wish for comfort and his insistence on declining treatments. Johnny's goals of care were switched to comfort, and he was discharged back to the long-term care facility where he died peacefully within 48 hours.

---

Johnny's story reveals contradictions not uncommonly seen in many persons with progressive life-threatening illnesses: not wanting to die, but no longer wanting to live in their current situation. His story illustrates several of the psychosocial issues outlined in Table 5.3. Johnny had multiple serious end-organ diseases: ESRD, chronic obstructive pulmonary disease, cirrhosis, and a suspected metastatic malignancy that complicated understanding the trajectory and symptom management given his ambivalence regarding goals of care. His manner of coping to avoid being "hassled" was challenged by a treatment required three times a week. His relationship with family was fragile and just reestablished after years of estrangement. Assuming that a family member who had not been in Johnny's life for years is in the best position to assume the responsibility of surrogate decision maker seems both unfair and unlikely to provide the most reliable "substituted" judgment. Johnny's behaviors were inconsistent with his words: his nonadherence to dialysis would likely shorten his life, but at the same time he wanted to be kept going. While Johnny had decisional capacity, before the delirium associated with uremia set in, he might have expressed his wishes for end-of-life care in an advance directive. This did not occur despite his social worker's encouragement to consider articulating his wishes.

Johnny also reminds us of the resilience of a black man who had no doubt experienced years of discrimination and acted in a manner that was consistent with what mattered to him.[68] Johnny may have been drawing on his faith, "an important and private" source of support. Many researchers and scholars have reported on the role of spirituality as source of comfort for the African American community.[16,68,69] Johnny died the way he wanted. However, for those taking care of Johnny, his nonadherence, reluctance to engage, and apparent ambivalence about goals of care presented a moral dilemma that required reflection and debriefing.

## Program-, Community-, and Policy-Level Approaches

Although there are no clinical practice guidelines developed specifically to define palliative care of the underserved, *Clinical Practice Guidelines for Quality Palliative Care* does serve as useful framework for developing and evaluating services to meet the unique needs of these populations.[70] In particular, preferred practices addressing social aspects of care (domain 4), spiritual, religious, and existential aspects of care (domain 5), and cultural aspects of care (domain 6) can be used to shape program development and service evaluation.

Two programs designed to meet the palliative care of the poor—a home care–based program in Hawaii[61] and a shelter-based program in Canada[60]—documented cost savings and favorable results for other quality indicators. These may serve as models for other communities with different needs and resources to consider in program development. Additionally, palliative care services in safety net hospitals have demonstrated improved family satisfaction and have increased the likelihood of patients and surrogate decision makers agreeing to DNR orders when the patient is seriously ill and unlikely to survive this intervention.[62,63]

Obviously, at the policy and community levels, stable housing is critical to providing a decent quality of life for any human. Researchers noted the benefits of supportive housing to minority elders in East Harlem, including better psychological outcomes and increased use of informal supports,[71] and to persons who were chronically homeless with severe alcohol problems in Seattle, which demonstrated cost savings.[72] Housing First is a policy advocated for the homeless and for professionals caring for them as the initial step in turning around the lives of homeless people with the hope preventing their premature death (http://www.endhomelessness.org/pages/housing_first). Advocating for housing for the urban poor and for the homeless is as critical as advocating for their preventive care, chronic disease management, symptom management, opportunities to articulate wishes about end-of-life care, spiritual care, and mental health and addiction services. Without safe housing, the opportunities for a "good enough" death may not be possible.

Several scholars have argued regarding the social justice implications of palliative and end-of-life care. Crawley noted that within the African American community, premature deaths have been associated with both individual and institutional injustices.[73] Racism, discrimination, health disparities, and research abuses such as Tuskegee have betrayed the trust of many African Americans and in part explained the determination among some to "go down fighting" rather than embrace some notion of a good death. The provocative essayist Krakauer warned that advocating for palliative care in situations in which disease-modifying therapies were standard of care for resourced communities or countries was unjust, unacceptable, and perhaps unethical.[74] His argument was based on concerns about global efforts to offer palliative care to persons suffering with cancer or HIV disease because the costs of disease therapies were exorbitant and unattainable by resource-strapped developing economies. The same argument could be made for the poor in the United States. Palliative care should not be promoted as a substitute for society's failure to provide all Americans, rich and poor alike, with their basic needs for food, clothing, shelter, education, employment, community, and promising futures. In that way, palliative care must be part of a healthcare system and social contract that include indicators of socioeconomic well-being alongside safe environments, food and shelter, meaningful employment, support for families and communities, health promotion, disease prevention, chronic disease management, and palliative care.

## Summary

Providing palliative care to the poor, especially the homeless, is extremely challenging. Treating comorbid illnesses and illnesses associated with poverty and clarifying the causes of presenting symptoms may seem almost impossible at times. Psychosocial risk factors and strained relationships with healthcare providers sometimes result in the client receiving futile or unwanted medical interventions at an advanced stage of illness. Clarifying with patients what constitutes a good death for them can be humbling when patients tell you they simply want to have shelter and to feel safe. Meeting the palliative care needs of this underserved population will require innovative practice and education models. To truly improve end-of-life care for the poor, nurses need to advocate for public policies that ensure access to safe and stable housing, health insurance, and client-centered, community-based primary care.[75]

## Acknowledgments

The author gratefully acknowledges the research and educational grant support of the American Cancer Society Doctoral Scholarship in Nursing;

National Institute of Nursing Research, Ruth L. Kirschstein National Research Service Award F31NR079923; Oncology Nursing Society (ONS) Foundation Small Research Grant Award; ONS Doctoral Scholarship; UCSF Alpha Eta Research Award, Sigma Theta Tau Chapter; and UCSF Graduate Student Research Award. She dedicates this chapter to the memory of Al, Tiffany, and Johnny—though they are no longer in this world, their stories and the stories of others like them continue to illuminate.

## References

1. Flaskerud JH, Winslow BJ. Conceptualizing vulnerable populations health-related research. *Nurs Res.* 1998;47(2):69–78.
2. Hughes A. Meeting the palliative care needs of the underserved. In: Dahlin CM, Lynch MT, eds. *Core Curriculum for the Advanced Practice Hospice and Palliative Care Registered Nurse*, Pittsburgh, PA: Hospice and Palliative Nurses Association; 2013:529–544.
3. Smedley BD, Stith AY, Nelson AR. *Unequal Treatment: Confronting Racial and Ethnic Disparities in Health Care.* Washington, DC: National Academy Press; 2003.
4. Koenig BA, Gates-Williams J. Understanding cultural difference in caring for dying patients. *West J Med.* 1995;163(3):244–249.
5. Freeman HP. Poverty, culture and social injustice: determinants of cancer disparities. *CA Cancer J Clin.* 2004;54(2):72–77.
6. Galea S, Tracy M, Hoggatt KJ, et al. Estimated deaths attributable to social Factors in the United States. *Am J Publ Health.* 2011;101(8):1456–1465.
7. Gibson R. Palliative care for the poor and disenfranchised: a view from the Robert Wood Johnson Foundation. J R Soc Med 2001;94:486–489.
8. Hughes A. Poverty and palliative care in the US: Issues facing the urban poor. *Int J Palliat Nurs.* 2005;11:6–13.
9. Hughes A. Meeting the palliative care needs of the underserved. In: Dahlin CM, Lynch MT, eds. *Core Curriculum for the Advanced Practice Hospice and Palliative Care Registered Nurse*, Pittsburgh, PA: Hospice and Palliative Nurses Association; 2013:529–544.
10. Hughes A, Davies B, Gudmundsdottir M. "Can you give me respect?" Experiences of the urban poor on a dedicated AIDS nursing home unit. *J Assoc Nurses AIDS Care.* 2008;19:342–356.
11. Hughes A, Gundmundsdottir M, Davies B. Everyday struggling to survive: experiences of the urban poor living with advanced cancer. *Oncol Nurs Forum.* 2007;34:1113–1118.
12. Moller DW. *Dancing with broken bones: portraits of death and dying among inner-city poor.* New York, NY: Oxford University Press; 2004.
13. Song J, Bartels DM, Ratner ER, et al. Dying on the streets: homeless persons' concerns and desires about end of life care. *J Gen Intern Med.* 2007;22(4):435–441.
14. Song J, Ratner ER, Bartels DM, et al. Experiences with and attitudes toward death and dying among homeless persons. *J Gen Intern Med.* 2007;22(4):427–434.
15. Lewis JM, DiGiacomo M, Currow DC, Davidson PM. Dying in the margins: understanding palliative care and socioeconomic deprivation in the developed world. *J Pain Symptom Manage.* 2011;42(1):105–118.

16. Dzul-Church V, Cimino JW, Adler SR, et al. "I'm sitting here by myself ...": experiences of patients with serious illness at an Urban Public Hospital. *J Palliat Med.* 2010;13(6):695–701.

17. Lyckholm LJ, Coyne PJ, Kreutzer KO, et al. Barriers to effective palliative care for low-income patients in late stages of cancer: report of a study and strategies for defining and conquering the barriers. *Nurs Clin North Am.* 2010;45(3):399–409.

18. Song J, Wall MM, Ratner ER, et al. Engaging homeless persons in end of life preparations. *J Gen Intern Med.* 2008;23(12):2031–2036; quiz 2037–2045.

19. Kushel MB, Miaskowski C. End-of-life care for homeless patients: "She says she is there to help me in any situation." *JAMA.* 2006;296(24):2959–2966.

20. Lewis JM, DiGiacomo M, Currow DC, Davidson PM. Dying in the margins: understanding palliative care and socioeconomic deprivation in the developed world. *J Pain Symptom Manage.* 2011;42(1):105–118.

21. Taipale V. Ethics and allocation of health resources: the influence of poverty on health. *Acta Oncol.* 1999;38:51–55.

22. Blacksher E. On being poor and feeling poor: low socioeconomic status and the moral self. *Theor Med Bioeth.* 2002;23:455–470.

23. Hughes AM. *"Can you give me respect?" Experiences of the urban poor with advanced disease.* San Francisco, CA: University of California San Francisco School of Nursing; 2007:202.

24. Aday LA. *At Risk in America: The Health and Health Care Needs of Vulnerable Populations.* 2nd ed. San Francisco: Jossey-Bass; 2001

25. DeNavas-Walt C, Proctor BD, Smith JC. Income, poverty, and health insurance coverage in the United States: 2011. *Curr Popul Rep.* 2012;Sept.:60–243.

26. Macartney S, Mykyta L. Poverty and shared households by state: 2011. *Am Commun Surv Briefs.* 2012;ACSBR/11-05.

27. National Coalition for the Homeless. *How Many People Experience Homelessness?* 2009. http://www.nationalhomeless.org/factsheets/How_Many.html. Accessed August 22, 2015.

28. Crawley J, Kane D, Atkinson-Plato L, et al. Needs of the hidden homeless—no longer hidden: a pilot study. *Public Health.* 2013;127(7):674–680.

29. Fellin P. The culture of homelessness. In: Manoleas P, ed. *Cross-Cultural Practice of Clinical Case Management in Mental Health.* New York, NY: Haworth Press; 1996:41–77.

30. Strechlow AJ, Amos-Jones T. The homeless as a vulnerable population. *Nurs Clin North Am.* 1999;34(2):261–274.

31. National Coalition for the Homeless. *Who Is Homeless?* 2009. http://www.nationalhomeless.org/factsheets/. Accessed September 12, 2015.

32. Lynch J, Smith GD, Harper S, Hillemeier M. Is income inequality a determination of population health? Pt 2. U.S. national and regional trends in income inequality and age- and cause-specific mortality. *Millbank Q.* 2004;82(2):355–400.

33. Horne BD, et al. Less affluent area of residence and lesser-insured status predict an increased risk of death or myocardial infarction after angiographic diagnosis of coronary disease. *Annu Epidemiol.* 2003;14:143–150.

34. Fang J, Alderman MH. Is geography destiny for patients in new york with myocardial infarction? *Am J Med.* 2003;115:448–453.

35. Hossain WA, Ehtesham MW, Salzman GA, et al. Healthcare access and disparities in chronic medical conditions in urban populations. *South Med J*. 2013;106(4):246–254.
36. Baggett TP, Hwang SW, O'Connell JJ, et al. Mortality among homeless adults in Boston: shifts in causes of death over a 15-year period. *JAMA*. 2013;173(3):189–195.
37. Patchell T. Nowhere to run: portraits of life on the street. *Turning Wheel: Journal of Socially Engaged Buddhism*. 1996:14–21.
38. Crawley LM. Racial, cultural, and ethnic factors influencing end-of-life care. *J Palliat Med*. 2005;8(Suppl 1):S58–69.
39. Hawkins NM, Jhund PS, McMurray JJ, Capewell S. Heart failure and socioeconomic status: accumulating evidence of inequality. *Eur J Heart Fail*. 2012;14(2):138–146.
40. Gordon EJ, Ladner DP, Caicedo JC, Franklin J. Disparities in kidney transplant outcomes: a review. *Semin Nephrol*. 2010;30(1):81–89.
41. Smith AK, Ladner D, McCarthy EP. Racial/ethnic disparities in liver transplant surgery and hospice use: parallels, differences, and unanswered questions. *Am J Hosp Palliat Care*. 2008;25(4):285–291.
42. Edwards TA, Jandorf L, Freemantle H, et al. Cancer care in East and Central Harlem: community partnership needs assessment. *J Cancer Educ*. 2013;28(1):171–178.
43. American Cancer Society. *Cancer Facts & Figures 2011*. Atlanta, GA: American Cancer Society; 2011.
44. Barnato AE, Anthony DL, Skinner J, et al. Racial and ethnic differences in preferences for end-of-life treatment. *J Gen Intern Med*. 2009;24(6):695–701.
45. Kiefer CW. *Health Work With the Poor: A Practical Guide*. New Brunswick, NJ: Rutgers University Press; 2000.
46. Bender M, Clarke E, Guilbe M, Selwyn PA. Missed opportunities in providing palliative care for the urban poor: a case discussion. *J Palliat Med*. 2013;16:587–590.
47. O'Connor PG, Selwyn PA, Schottenfeld RS. Medical care for injection drug users with human immunodeficiency syndrome. *N Engl J Med*. 1994;331:450–459.
48. Centers for Disease Control and Prevention. Opioids drive continued increase in drug overdose deaths. 2013. http://www.cdc.gov/media/releases/2013/p0220_drug_overdose_deaths.html. Accessed August 23, 2015.
49. Morrison RS, Wallenstein S, Natale DK, et al. "We don't carry that"—Failure of pharmacies in predominantly nonwhite neighborhoods to stock opioid analgesics. *N Engl J Med*. 2000;342:1023–1026.
50. Soares LGL. Poor social condition, criminality and urban violence: unmentioned barriers for effective cancer pain control at the end of life. *J Pain Symptom Manage*. 2003;26(2):693–695.
51. Kircher S, Zacny J, Apfelbaum SM, et al. Understanding and treating opioid addiction in a patient with cancer pain. *J Pain*. 2011;12(10):1025–1031.
52. Newshan G, Staats JA. Evidence-based pain guidelines in HIV care. *J Assoc Nurses AIDS Care*. 2013;24(1 Suppl):S112–126.
53. Passik SD. Issues in long-term opioid therapy: unmet needs, risks, and solutions. *Mayo Clin Proc*. 2009;84(7):593–601.

54. Chou R, Fanciullo GJ, Fine PG, et al. Opioids for chronic noncancer pain: prediction and identification of aberrant drug-related behaviors: a review of the evidence for an American Pain Society and American Academy of Pain Medicine clinical practice guideline. *J Pain*. 2009;10(2):131–146.

55. Miaskowski C, Penko JM, Guzman D, et al. Occurrence and characteristics of chronic pain in a community-based cohort of indigent adults living with HIV infection. *J Pain*. 2011;12(9):1004–1116.

56. Guidelines for the use of antivirals in HIV-1– Infected adults and adolescents. https://aidsinfo.nih.gov/contentfiles/lvguidelines/adultadolescentgl.pds. Accessed September 12, 2015.

57. Bangsberg D, Tulsky JP, Hecht FM, Moss AR. Protease inhibitors in the homeless. *JAMA*. 1997;278:63–65.

58. United Way. *The Bottom Line: Setting the Real Standard for Bay Area Working Families*. 2004, San Francisco, CA: United Way of Bay Area; 2004:28.

59. Hughes A. Poor, homeless and underserved populations. In: Ferrell BR, Coyle N, eds. *Oxford Textbook of Palliative Nursing*. New York, NY: Oxford University Press; 2010:745–755.

60. Podymow T, Turnbull J, Coyle D. Shelter-based palliative care for the homeless terminally ill. *Palliat Med*. 2006;20(2):81–86.

61. Fernandes R, Braun KL, Ozawa J, et al. Home-based palliative care services for underserved populations. *J Palliat Med*. 2010;13(4):413–419.

62. Kaufer M, Murphy P, Barker K, Mosenthal A. Family satisfaction following the death of a loved one in an inner city MICU. *Am J Hosp Palliat Care*. 2008;25(4):318–325.

63. Sacco J, Carr DR, Viola D. The effects of the palliative medicine consultation on the DNR status of African Americans in a safety-net hospital. *Am J Hosp Palliat Care*. 2013;30(4):363–369.

64. Tarzian AJ, Neal MT, O'Neil JA. Attitudes, experiences, and beliefs affecting end-of-life decision-making among homeless individuals. *J Palliat Med*. 2005;8(1):36–48.

65. Sudore RL, Landefeld CS, Barnes DE, et al. An advance directive redesigned to meet the literacy level of most adults: a randomized trial. *Patient Educ Couns*. 2007;69(1-3):165–195.

66. Dula A, Williams S. When race matters. *Clin Geriatr Med*. 2005;21(1):239–253, xi.

67. Davis E, Tamayo A, Fernandez A. "Because somebody cared about me. That's how it changed things": homeless, chronically ill patients' perspectives on case management. *PLoS One*. 2012;7(9):e45980.

68. Teti M, Martin AE, Renade R, et al. "I'm a keep rising. I'm a keep going forward, regardless": exploring Black men's resilience amid sociostructural challenges and stressors. *Qual Health Res*. 2012;22(4):524–533.

69. Born W, Greiner KA, Sylvia E, et al. Knowledge, attitudes, and beliefs about end-of-life care among inner-city African Americans and Latinos. *J Palliat Med*. 2004;7(2):247–256.

70. National Consensus Project. *Clinical Practice Guidelines for Quality Palliative Care*. 3rd ed. Pittsburgh, PA: National Consensus Project for Quality Palliative Care; 2013.

71. Cleak H, Howe JL. Social networks and use of social supports of minority elders inn East Harlem. *Social Work Health Care*. 2003;38(1):19–38.

72. Larimer ME, Malone DK, Garner MD, et al. Health care and public service use and costs before and after provision of housing for chronically homeless persons with severe alcohol problems. *JAMA*. 2009;301(13):1349–1357.
73. Crawley LM. Palliative care in African American communities. *J Palliat Med*. 2002;5(5):775–779.
74. Krakauer EL. Just palliative care: responding responsibly to the suffering of the poor. J Pain Symptom Manage. 2008;36(5):505–512.
75. Patchell T. Suggestions for effective outreach. San Francisco, CA: San Francisco Department of Public Health, Homeless Death Prevention Project; 1997.

# Appendix

# Self-Assessment Test Questions

Nessa Coyle

## Questions

1. A 75-year-old widower with end-stage congestive heart failure expresses a desire to hasten his death. His three children live out of state and rarely call or visit. He experiences severe dyspnea and states, "I can't stand it anymore." The nurse's BEST initial response should be which of the following?
   A. "May I call your children to discuss this further?"
   B. "You seem depressed to me, and an antidepressant may help."
   C. "What is the most difficult thing about your situation?"
   D. "We can effectively treat your shortness of breath."

2. A family desires hospice care for their mother with end-stage breast cancer and requests the words "hospice" or "cancer" not be used when talking to her. Which of the following is the *most* appropriate nursing action?
   A. Request a consultation from the ethics committee.
   B. Discuss with the family the basis for their request.
   C. Delay hospice admission until the family meets with a social worker.
   D. Explain to the family that the patient should be made aware of the prognosis.

3. At the request of the family, a physician orders intravenous fluids for an elderly patient who is in the final stage of Alzheimer's disease. The nurse's *most* appropriate response is which of the following?
   A. Initiate the intravenous hydration as ordered.
   B. Initiate a trial of intravenous fluids for a period of 72 hours.
   C. Discuss with the family the benefits and burdens of hydration.
   D. Discuss with the interdisciplinary team the physician's orders because the patient may no longer be appropriate for hospice.

4. The President's Commission for the Study of Ethical Problems concluded which of the following regarding giving opioids to relieve the suffering of a terminally ill patient?
   A. It is for the family's comfort rather than the patient's.
   B. It is acceptable even when the drugs may suppress breathing.
   C. It is acceptable, but not to the point of suppressing breathing.
   D. It has not been fully explored ethically and should, therefore, be avoided.

5. A patient's physician has ordered a placebo by injection on a routine basis. The nurse should do which of the following?
   A. Decline to administer the placebo.
   B. Teach the family to administer the placebo.
   C. Assess the patient's response to the placebo.
   D. Recognize that psychological pain is often relieved by placebos.

## Answers

1. C
2. B
3. C
4. B
5. A

# Index

References to tables and boxes are denoted by an italicized *t* and *b*.

advance care
 planning, 5–6
 documentation, 6
 ethics of, 7–8
Affordable Care Act, 101
aggression, psychotic
 disorders, 73–74
agitation, artificial
 hydration, 55
Alzheimer's disease, case
 study, 48
American Academy
 of Hospice and
 Palliative Medicine
 (AAHPM), 16*b*, 20,
 40, 41*b*, 42
American Cancer
 Society, 96
American Nurses
 Association
 (ANA), 22, 23, 33*t*
American Society for
 Pain Management
 Nursing, 16*b*, 33*t*
amyotrophic lateral
 sclerosis (ALS), 36,
 49, 57*t*
ANH. See artificial
 nutrition and
 hydration (ANH)
anorexia, 99
 artificial hydration, 52
 artificial
 nutrition, 49, 50, 51
anticonvulsants, 79*b*
artificial hydration, 52–56
 agitation, 55
 benefits and
 burdens, 53–54
 confusion, 55
 dehydration, 54–55
 delirium, 55
 fluid retention, 54–55
 methods of
 administration, 52–53
 myoclonus, 55
 potential
 complications, 53*t*
 quality of life, 55–56
 survival benefit, 55

thirst and dry
 mouth, 55
artificial nutrition, 48–52
 anorexia, 50
 benefits and
 burdens, 49–50
 cachexia, 50
 complications of enteral
 support, 50*t*
 dysphagia, 50
 hunger, 50–51
 malnutrition, 50
 methods of
 administration, 49
 pressure ulcers, 51
 quality of life, 51–52
 survival time, 51
artificial nutrition
 and hydration
 (ANH), 7, 11, 47
 case study, 14–15, 48
 cultural issues, 58–59
 decision making, 57–61
 engaging in
 conversations
 about, 60
 ethical issues, 57, 58*t*
 ethics of, 12–15
 family concerns, 13
 financial implications, 14
 guidelines, 57*t*
 hydration, 52–56
 implementing
 decision, 61
 legal precedent, 58
 nutrition, 48–52
 patients making
 informed
 choices, 60–61
 position statements and
 guidelines, 56–57
 position statements
 from professional
 organizations, 16*b*
 religious issues, 58–59,
 59*t*, 60*t*
assistance in dying, 30
 access, 35–37
 alternatives
 to, 40, 42–43

ethical and legal
 issues, 31–35
 nurses and, 38–39
 nurses' responses to
 requests, 40, 41*b*
 palliative care and
 requests for, 29–31
 perspectives of families
 and healthcare
 providers, 37
 principle of double
 effect, 31
 reasons for
 request, 37–38
 withholding or
 withdrawing
 life-sustaining
 measures, 30–31
assisted suicide, 15, 17
automatic internal
 cardiofibrillators
 (AICDs), 17–18

Belgium, euthanasia, 32
benzodia-
 zepines, 19, 52, 79
bipolar disease, 77–81
 case study, 80–81
 communication
 issues, 79–80
 nonpharmacologic
 treatment, 79
 pharmacologic
 treatment, 78–79
 treatment
 of, 78–79, 79*b*
breast cancer, metastatic,
 to brain, 56
Buddhism, artificial
 hydration and
 nutrition (AHN), 59*t*
burnout, 23

cachexia
 artificial nutrition, 50
 cancer, 49
calcium channel
 blockers, 79*b*
cancer
 cachexia, 49

# Index

cancer (Cont.)
  poverty and, 97b
  suicide, 36
  see also case studies
capacity
  bipolar disorder, 78
  proxy decision making, 10
  serious mental illness, 72–73
cardiac assistive devices, hastening death, 17–19
cardiopulmonary resuscitation (CPR), 8–9, 12t, 21
case studies
  feeding tube decisions, 4–5
  hospice patient and suicide interest, 43
  patient with AIDS-related non-Hodgkin's lymphoma, 99
  patient with Alzheimer's and progressive dementia, 48
  patient with bipolar disease, 80–81
  patient with colon cancer, 84–85
  patient with end-stage renal disease (ESRD), 107–8
  patient with lung cancer, 95
  patient with metastatic breast cancer to brain, 56
  patient with schizophrenia, 76–77
  withdrawal of life support, 14–15
Catholicism, artificial hydration and nutrition (AHN), 59t
Centers for Disease Control and Prevention, 100
central nervous system, lung cancer metastasis to, 95
Clinical Practice Guidelines for Quality Palliative Care, 8
clozapine, 71t, 76
Code of Ethics for Nurses, American Nurses Association (ANA), 22, 23
cognitive-behavioral therapy (CBT), 71, 79, 82, 83

colon cancer, case study, 84–85
communication issues
  advance care planning, 6–7
  bipolar disorder, 79–80
  difficult-to-engage clients, 105b
  palliative sedation, 42
  psychotic disorders, 74–75
  requests for assisted dying, 40
  serious mental illness, 69
compassion fatigue, 23–24
competency
  proxy decision making, 10
  serious mental illness, 72–73
confusion, artificial hydration, 55
coping strategies, 24

death. See hastening death
Death with Dignity Act
  Oregon, 32, 35–37, 38
  Washington State, 15, 35, 39
decision making, proxy, 10–11
dehydration, artificial hydration, 54–55
delirium, artificial hydration, 55
dementia, case study, 48
destination therapy, 18
Diagnostic and Statistical Manual of Mental Disorders, fifth edition (DSM-5), 78
do-not-attempt-resuscitation (DNAR)
  ethics of, 7
  orders, 8–10
  proxy decision making, 11
  rationale, 9–10
dry mouth, artificial hydration, 55
durable power of attorney for healthcare (DPAHC), 6, 11
dysphagia, artificial nutrition, 50

end-of-life care, serious mental illness and, 68–69
end-stage renal disease (ESRD), 96, 107–8

ethics
  advance care planning, 5–6
  of care, 3
  case study, 4–5
  common dilemmas, 4–5
  compassion fatigue, 23–24
  coping strategies, 24
  definition, 2
  feminist, 3
  goal setting, 5–6
  moral distress, 24
  narrative, 3
  nursing issues, 22–24
  preventive, 6–8
  process, 3–11
  serious mental illness at end of life, 72–73
  steps of ethical problem solving, 4b
euthanasia, 15, 17, 32

families
  artificial nutrition and hydration, 13
  assistance in dying, 37
  serious mental illness (SMI), 75–76
feminist ethics, 3
fluid retention, artificial hydration, 54–55
futility, 20–22

Gilligan, Carol, 3
Global Burden of Disease Study, 67
goal setting, ethics of, 5–6

hastening death
  assisted suicide, 15, 17
  cardiac assistive devices, 17–19
  euthanasia, 15, 17
  futility, 20–22
  palliative sedation concerns, 19–20
  position statements from professional organizations, 16b
  principle of double effect, 20
healthcare providers, assistance in dying, 37
health care proxy, 6
Hinduism, artificial hydration and nutrition (AHN), 59t
homelessness
  case study, 95

death of homeless people, 94–95
definition, 92
health problems associated with, 93t, 93–94
prevalence of, 92
Hospice and Palliative Nurses Association (HPNA), 16b, 20, 33t, 34t
Hunger, artificial nutrition, 50–51
hydration. See artificial hydration

incompetency, 10
Islam, artificial hydration and nutrition (AHN), 59t

Joint Commission on Accreditation of Healthcare Organizations, 24
Judaism, artificial hydration and nutrition (AHN), 60t

left ventricular assistive devices (LVADs), 17, 18
life support, case study for withdrawal of, 14–15
lung cancer, case study, 95
Luxembourg, euthanasia, 32

malnutrition, artificial nutrition, 50
medical futility, 20–22
medical orders for life-sustaining treatment (MOLST), 7–8
medication
 antipsychotic, 71t
 antiretroviral (ARV), 99, 100–102
 assisted dying, 30, 32, 33t, 38–40
 bipolar disorder, 78–79, 79b
 palliative sedation, 19
 psychotic disorders, 70–72
 right to refuse, 72
 schizophrenia, 76–77
mental illness
 barriers to care for patients with, 69
 patients with serious, 67–68

see also serious mental illness (SMI)
MOLST. See medical orders for life-sustaining treatment (MOLST)
Montana, assisted suicide, 35
mood stabilizers, 78, 79b
moral distress, 23, 24
moral fatigue, 23
moral reasoning, 2–3
myoclonus, artificial hydration, 55

narrative ethics, 3
National Alliance on Mental Illness (NAMI), 75
National Coalition for the Homeless, 92
National Consensus Project for Quality Palliative Care, 8
National Hospice and Palliative Care Organization (NHPCO), 16b, 20
Netherland, assisted suicide, 32, 36
new stealth euthanasia, 30
non-Hodgkin's lymphoma, 99
nursing responsibilities
 assisted dying and, 38–39
 hastening death, 17
 preventive ethics, 8
nutrition. See artificial nutrition

Oncology Nursing Society, 16b, 34t, 40, 111
Oregon
 Death with Dignity Act, 32, 35–37, 38
 end-of-life care, 7, 38, 40
 physician-assisted suicide, 15, 17
 POLST Paradigm, 7
Oregon Nurses Association, assisted dying, 34t, 40

pacemakers, 17–18
palliative care
 assistance in dying, 29–31
 barriers and challenges, 102–4
 ethical considerations, 1

evidence-based, for urban poor, 104
personality disorders and, 81–85
program-, community- and policy-level approaches for poor, 109–10
psychosocial challenges in providing, to urban poor, 103t
palliative sedation, 19
 alternative to assisted dying, 42
 hastening death, 19–20
 position statements from professional organizations, 16b
palliative sedation to unconsciousness (PSU), 19, 20
Patient Self-Determination Act (PSDA), 7
percutaneous endoscopic gastrostomy (PEG), 13, 48, 49
personality disorders
 case study, 84–85
 cluster A, 81–82
 cluster B, 82
 cluster C, 82
 communication issues, 83–84
 palliative care, 68, 81–85
 treatment of, 82–83
physician-assisted death, 32, 37, 41b
physician-assisted suicide (PAS), 15, 16b, 32, 34t, 35–36
physician orders for life-sustaining treatment (POLST), 7–8, 38
poverty, 89–91
 assessment considerations, 106–9
 cancer and, 97b
 case study, 95, 99, 107–8
 clinical interventions, 104–6
 clinical presentations of advanced disease in poor, 98–99, 100–102
 epidemiology of, 91–92
 health problems associated with, 93–94
 insights about dying poor, 98b

poverty (*Cont.*)
life-threatening illness and quality of life, 95–98
program-, community- and policy-level approaches, 109–10
states with rates exceeding national average, 91*t*
pressure ulcers, 51
preventive ethics, 6–8
principle of double effect, 20, 31
progressive dementia, case study, 48
Protestant, artificial hydration and nutrition (AHN), 60*t*
proxy decision making, 10–11, 12*t*
psychotic disorders
aggression, 73–74
antipsychotic medications, 71*t*
case study of schizophrenia, 76–77
communication and, 74–75
family issues, 75–76
nonpharmacologic treatment, 71–72
pharmacologic treatment, 70–71
schizophrenia and, 69–77
treatment of, 70–72

quality of life
artificial hydration, 55–56
artificial nutrition, 51–52
poverty and life-threatening illness, 95–98

religious beliefs, artificial hydration and nutrition (AHN), 59*t*, 60*t*

schizophrenia
antipsychotic medications, 71*t*
case study, 76–77
nonpharmacologic treatment, 71–72
pharmacologic treatment, 70–71
psychotic disorders, 69–77
treatment of, 70–72
self-assessment test, 117–18

serious mental illness (SMI), 67–68, 69
advance directives, 72
aggression, 73–74
capacity and competency, 72–73
and end-of-life care, 68–69, 85
ethical issues in caring for, 72–73
family issues, 75–76
right to refuse medication, 72
survival
artificial hydration, 55
artificial nutrition, 51
Switzerland, euthanasia, 32

thirst, artificial hydration, 55

Vermont State Nurses' Association (VSNA), assisted dying, 34*t*
Veterans Administration, 6, 69
voluntary refusal of food and fluids (VSED), 42
vulnerable population, 89

Washington State, Death with Dignity Act, 15, 35, 39

www.ingramcontent.com/pod-product-compliance
Ingram Content Group UK Ltd.
Pitfield, Milton Keynes, MK11 3LW, UK
UKHW021258180426
11947UKWH00015B/910